THE 7 PILLARS
MANIFESTATION

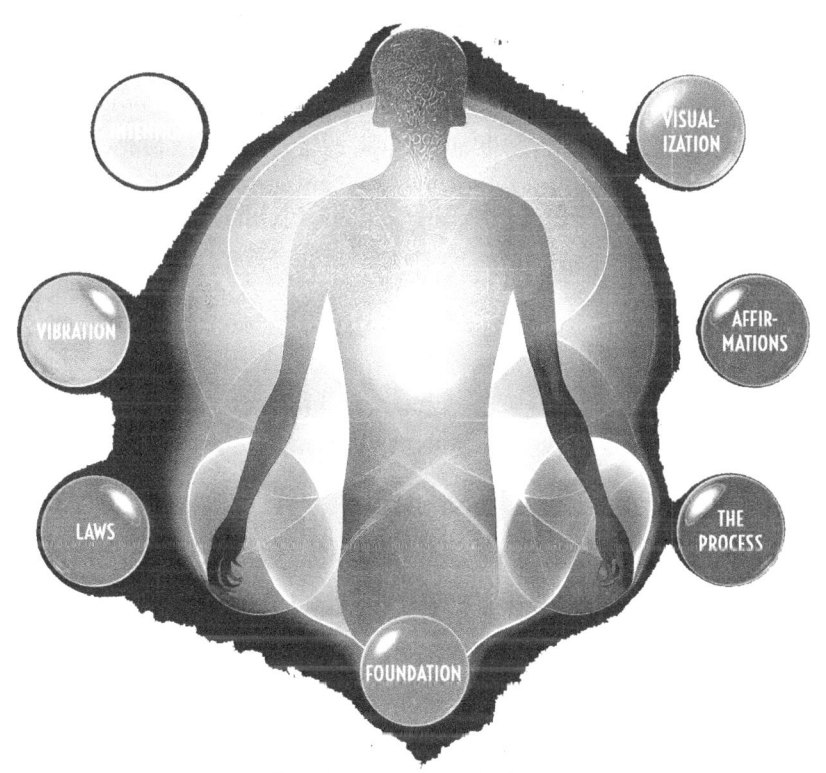

- VISUALIZATION
- AFFIRMATIONS
- THE PROCESS
- FOUNDATION
- LAWS
- VIBRATION

107 Techniques & Clues
to Create the Life You Want with the Power of Your Mind. Manifest Happiness, Money, Success, and Love by Raising Your Vibration and Energy

INGRID CLARKE

© **Copyright 2023 - All rights reserved.**

The content contained within this book may not be reproduced, duplicated, or transmitted without direct written permission from the author or the publisher.

Under no circumstances will any blame or legal responsibility be held against the publisher, or author, for any damages, reparation, or monetary loss due to the information contained within this book, either directly or indirectly.

Legal Notice:

This book is copyright protected. It is only for personal use. You cannot amend, distribute, sell, use, quote, or paraphrase any part of the content within this book without the consent of the author or publisher.

Disclaimer Notice:

Please note the information contained within this document is for educational and entertainment purposes only. All effort has been executed to present accurate, up-to-date, reliable, and complete information. No warranties of any kind are declared or implied. Readers acknowledge that the author is not engaged in the rendering of legal, financial, medical, or professional advice. The content within this book has been derived from various sources. Please consult a licensed professional before attempting any techniques outlined in this book.

By reading this document, the reader agrees that under no circumstances is the author responsible for any losses, direct or indirect, that are incurred as a result of the use of the information contained within this document, including, but not limited to, errors, omissions, or inaccuracies.

Table of Contents

Introduction 5

Pillar One: Foundation 11
    What Is Manifestation? 12
    The Origin 13
    The Science Behind It 16
    Becoming a Self-Fulfilling Prophecy 17

Pillar Two: Laws 21
    Law of Oneness 22
    Law of Vibration 23
    Law of Correspondence 24
    Law of Attraction 25
    Law of Action 27
    Law of Perpetual Transmutation of Energy 28
    Law of Cause and Effect 31
    Law of Compensation 33
    The Law of Relativity 34
    Law of Polarity 36
    Law of Rhythm 37
    Law of Gender 38

Pillar Three: Vibration 41
    What Is Vibrational Energy? 41
    What Are Vibrational Beings? 43

    Connection Between Thoughts, Behaviors, and Vibrations........44
    Raising Your Vibration 51

Pillar Four: Intention.. 67
    Intention Manifestation 68
    Setting Intentions.. 72

Pillar Five: Visualization 79
    Power of Visualization 80
    Multi-Sensory Visualization 83
    Practicing Visualization 84

Pillar Six: Affirmations.. 89
    The Power of Affirmations 90
    What Are Affirmations?... 99

Pillar Seven: The Process 105
    Identify and Clarify 106
    Ask the Universe 109
    Take Inspired Action 110
    Trust the Journey.. 110
    Release Attachment 111
    Be Grateful for What You Receive 112
    Watch Your Energy... 114
    Let Go of Limiting Beliefs... 116

Conclusion 119

Glossary 123

References 127

Introduction

Something in life has you feeling overwhelmed and wanting to see change. Yet, you never lost faith that the universe was generous because beneath all your triumphs and failings lies the power of your mind. And regardless of how hard life may seem, you always find the strength and courage to push on and continue striving for something greater. Perhaps, it was because you are aware that beyond the horizon lies a dream that can be pursued, regardless of age. Or deep inside your subconscious is an abundance of knowledge, power, wisdom, and all you need to create a life far more extraordinary than what you already have. Tapping into this possibility will lead you to achieve abundance in life. Likewise, it can help you ask the universe for what you truly want and propel your path to fulfillment.

Stress is an integral part of modern life. From our jobs to our businesses, on the way to work or even home, we stress daily as a form of survival. Growing up in a Scandinavian family with pagan roots, I understand how to face and deal with various hard situations, such as chronic stress or illness, without needing medication. In fact, I have gone through a great deal of exhaustion and stress in my life. Drawing from medical, metaphysical, and occult knowledge I have gained from research, I aim to share my understanding and experiences with those seeking transformation or relief. These years of study have imparted me with profound wisdom that can help anyone going through a difficult journey find comfort and hope for the future.

It is no secret that we possess great power in our minds, and it is our right to use it to create whatever we want. All we must do is align our minds with our dreams and put in the effort to make them come true. It is neither a game nor a celestial mystery; it is reality. This is our chance to demonstrate that if we set our minds on something, visualize it thoroughly, and take the appropriate steps; we can manifest it into reality.

With incredible gifts to do whatever we desire, it can be easy to get stuck in a negative spiral. Frustration sets in when things do not turn out as expected, and life can feel like an uphill battle. But with the help of our minds, we can learn how to use these gifts for good, turning our mindset around so that it works for us rather than against us. Reading this book offers a unique solution to shifting your mentality from a place of negativity, even if you feel overwhelmed or unable to manifest the life of your dreams. It provides the essential steps to reframe your ideas and create lasting change within yourself. Likewise, in this book, you can learn how to take control of your life by understanding the seven pillars of manifestation that can influence how energy and vibrations shape reality. Additionally, it provides insight into the theories, strategies, and advice for living abundantly, joyfully, and gloriously.

Overall, this book provides a simple yet powerful and unique approach to manifestation, which starts by delving into fundamental aspects such as the practice's science, history, and definition. This pillar will help you gain insight into the concept of manifestation, regardless of your experience level. Understanding this foundation helps to equip you for success as you move on with the other pillars.

For the following pillar, we will dive deeper into the laws and principles that help open your eyes to a mental and spiritual capacity. They will teach you how to design and create your reality consciously. Plus, you will have the chance to tap into the infinite intelligence and power within yourself and the universe. As a beginner, these pillars have the information you need to start.

- **Pillar II:** Understanding the universal laws and how they impact your life.
- **Pillar III:** Delves into how to raise the vibration and manifest your desires.
- **Pillars IV and V:** Explain the power of intention and visualization.
- **Pillar VI:** Examines the impact that affirmations have on you, your relationships, and your spiritual creator.
- **Pillar VII:** Outlines a seven-step framework for creating a beautiful and extraordinary life.

I was able to discover the potential of my mind and make huge strides in life. Now, it is an honor to pass down these invaluable tools and bestow their power onto you. Through applying these methods, I've seen challenges become mere obstacles and overcome them with grace, leading to new heights in my journey. Not to mention, these very methods assist celebrities in manifesting their dreams, such as:

- Jim Carrey used the power of visualization to transform his life from a janitor to an A-list actor

- Lady Gaga used the power of affirmation to become famous, even before people knew her name.
- Oprah Winfrey believed she would land a lead role in a movie she auditioned for at the start of her fame and fortune. She harnessed the power of clarity, universal trust, and gratitude for visualizing what she wanted and got the part.

Hence, this book offers an opportunity to manifest and reclaim control of your life. You can direct the power of your mind and build a success story unique to you, your goals, and your dreams. By exploring manifestations' common principles and practices, you will access greater pleasure, serenity, abundance, and empowerment. With these tools, you can craft your best life with healing and self-mastery as a guide. No matter where you are on your journey, this book offers a blueprint to help unlock what lies ahead.

Subsequently, the techniques and strategies you are about to read are proven to yield incredible results for people who want to tap into the healing power of manifestation. Each pillar in this book will teach you the different theories and techniques you can use in your spiritual journey to recognize your immense power to shift your life in the direction you want. I implore you to use the knowledge and strategies gained from this book to seize power. Remember, *knowledge is far more priceless when it is shared and acted upon.* Therefore, take substantial steps towards utilizing these teachings in your life; reap the rewards of realizing the greatness of realization.

Empower yourself with the knowledge you have and take action. With this, you will be closer to manifesting prosperity and abundance in your life. Aside from that, this provides easy access to information on manifestation, regardless of their physical, mental, or emotional state. And with the right mindset and perspective, you can turn things around, no matter what you face.

As you move forward with this book, please keep this in mind: *There is powerful energy already inherent to you.* You have the extraordinary capability of transforming your life using the power of your mind. Reach within yourself, tap into that energy, and use it to draw upon the universal laws. With this knowledge, you control your destiny. Likewise, you can manifest happiness, money, success, love, freedom, or whatever abundance you desire. Allow all these beautiful things to enter your life, embrace this power, and see how far it takes you.

No doubt, your life is on the cusp of a transformation as you have already taken the first step to bringing your dreams into reality—opening this book and beginning to read. Now, what happens next is entirely up to you.

Pillar One
Foundation

To manifest your goals and dreams, it is essential to construct a strong foundation. This applies to any pursuit we make as the foundation is an integral part of success. In this case, if you wish to see your dreams come true through manifestation, you need to acquire a comprehensive knowledge of its fundamentals, such as *"Why it exists?"*, *"Where its origin lies?"* and *"Why can countless people attest to its impact on their life?"* Understanding these fundamentals must be established before anything else can fall into place; hence, they form the first piece of the puzzle when entering the field of manifestation.

Once you comprehend the basics, you will realize how imperative it is to align your thoughts positively and be able to envision what you wish for, as manifestation can influence your life in unique ways. But without this foundation, you will begin your journey on rocky ground, and it will feel like such. Clarity will also be non-existent, and you will go back and forth, confused, and distracted, believing that manifestation does not work. Likewise, you will be stuck in a skeptic's mind frame, encountering feelings of stagnation, loss, and difficulty, asking yourself why it is so.

As such, this pillar will help set you up on the right foot. From the get-go, it will open your mind to the unique possibilities of manifestation. It can be a powerful tool to help you navigate challenges, opening doors that once felt sealed shut because of mistrust, lack of familiarity with the vision, or focusing on the struggle instead of the miracles of changing your outlook. Nevertheless, this pillar is here to help broaden your mental outlook and well-being.

What Is Manifestation?

According to Oprah Daily, Angelina Lombardo, a coach, and author, defines manifestation as *"making everything you want to feel and experience a reality via your thoughts, actions, beliefs, and emotions."* In other words, manifestation is the process in which you harness the power of your subconscious and align its energy with that of your goals and dreams to make them a reality. And instead of referring to the act of manifestation as 'harnessing,' think of it as a way to influence the power of your thoughts to achieve positive and empowered feelings, bringing in the energy of all you desire. Through this process, you can control your mind to create an atmosphere for these things to manifest.

Everyone can make their dreams come true. To some degree, we are constantly manifesting our reality, sometimes without even being aware. Our thoughts are potent and can help us achieve what we aspire to. Now, reflect on what is currently in your life. *How would you describe it? Is it encouraging? Difficult? Positive? Negative? Plentiful or lacking?* No matter how your life looks, know that it can always change for the better. If you are going through a tough time, try to see it as an opportunity. These challenges make us stronger and more capable of enduring hardship. Besides, manifesting is all about claiming our power. As you take action to create the life you want, ensure you are honoring your energy, owning up to any mistakes, and making choices that will allow you to move forward. It is also about the courage to choose something different if our actions are not working. Regardless, *what manifests in your life depends on your choices.*

However, remember that saying that you want something and genuinely meaning it is two different things. Many people can say they want a luxurious home or an exotic vacation, but when it comes to making these things happen, *you must be emotionally invested in them.* Feeling like there is no other option but to make your dreams a reality is what manifestation is all about. In a Google search, manifestation is defined as *something you embody.* The word embodiment could be used to describe the process of manifestation well. For manifestation to work in your life, you must feel what you intend to manifest. Believe that your manifestational dreams are meant for you to live in this lifetime, and you will stop at nothing to make them happen. As such, when you think of this innate urge to manifest your dream home or more money in your bank account, your drive and determination awaken, and things shift in your body, mind, and spirit. Then, your energy becomes infectious to the universe, and you attract abundance into your life.

The Origin

> *"All that we are is a result of what we have thought."*
>
> *–Buddha*

There are many people new to manifestation who believe that it is a relatively recent discovery. A taboo topic of magic and spirituality combined. Some have even described it as "hocus pocus witchcraft" or a journey where you create magic spells. But this is not the case. To begin your manifestation journey, you must understand its true origins. As such, you must know where it came from, how it started, and the like.

Manifestation has been around for centuries, even if it was not given the name yet. In fact, it did not become popular recently simply because someone thought it would be cool, as its origin can be traced back far before that. While the term might be new, the concept of manifestation certainly is not. Jesus speaks about manifestation many times in the bible when he talks about having unlimited power to give you what you need and wants as long as you put your trust and faith in him. For instance, 1 Corinthians 3:13 talks about how "each one's work will be made to manifest," Matthew 7:7 says, "ask, and you shall receive," and 2 Corinthians 5:7 says, "live by faith, not by sight." Many other scriptures also reference manifestation and the idea that we can manifest anything we want as long as we have faith.

What you think is powerful shapes your life and destiny. Through the practice of Hinduism, such as Kundalini yoga and the seven chakras, individuals can awaken their manifestational senses and intuition to gain insight into their true selves, allowing them to control their lives. Besides, far before we, as a human race, ever stepped foot on the earth, the concept of manifestation had already been born; *consider it a notion that has existed for ages and prevails even today.* As we grew up, we began to form our ideas and conclusions about the manifestation journey while staying within the vicinity of the original concept. Take the Law of Attraction as an example, a concept that has become familiar to many, leading to the introduction of other spiritual laws and teachings. It has been put forward that the Law of Attraction and its idea of *'like attracts like'* have persistently been at the core of how our life plays out.

So, has it only been a few decades since manifestation started existing in new-age spirituality? No, it has been many centuries since the dawn of time. By the 19th century, a Russian author named Helena Petrovna Blavatsky began introducing manifestation to the public. She wrote a book called *The Secret Doctrine*, exploring religious doctrines and speaking of our power to shape our reality. Likewise, she said that letting go of any negative thoughts and beliefs holding us back could make our dreams a reality. By pushing past these old hindrances, we can manifest anything we desire.

Thomas Troward, a 19th-century scholar and author, believed that the power of our mind could manifest what we think about into our reality. He thought whatever we immerse ourselves in, be it good or bad, would become an integral part of us. Meanwhile, his ideas toward manifestation, such as his influence on the Law of Cause and Effect, were known to have inspired the movie, *The Secret*. Troward believed that *"our mind is a center of divine operations"* and that *"the subconscious mind accepts uncritically whatever suggestion may be impressed upon it, and works out in great fidelity whatever may logically follow from the suggestion"* (n.d).

Ancient theologians and authors, who have studied spiritual and religious doctrines for many years, came to a similar conclusion about the way our minds interact with the laws of the universe; *a new-age university professor did not introduce this manifestation in our time but instead had existed for a long time.*

The Science Behind It

When we think about scientific procedures and process, scientist is passionate about experimentation. They will take an idea and mesh various substances together with a vision to form something. Yet, some scientists, like Alexander Fleming, would go on to create tangible things by mistake. In the early 1900s, Fleming was experimenting in his lab when he decided to pause his work to go on vacation. Upon his return, he noticed mold and bacteria growing in the dish he was working on because it was left slightly open. This mold became the development of penicillin, which is a common drug used today to counteract various infections.

Manifestation is like working in a laboratory of the mind. Establishing our goals and taking action to make them a reality requires a strong, unwavering faith that we can change our lives if we genuinely believe it is possible. We must have the conviction that this is possible and then take the necessary steps to make it happen. Likewise, translating thoughts into tangible, physical creations is all about doing whatever it takes to make it happen. This concept relates to taking action and pushing ourselves toward our goals. It takes hard work, stamina, complete dedication to our craft, and keeping our eye on the prize. Like Thomas Edison creating the light bulb, it took him and his team over 3,000 tries of trial and error to form the first light bulb that worked.

Many scientists have also studied the brain and its extraordinary capabilities. They have concluded that by the time we hit 20 years old, our brains have accumulated ten times more knowledge than the Encyclopedia Britannica. That means we have incredible power within us to visualize our dreams and make them a reality simply by shifting our mindset and taking consistent, inspired action toward our goals.

Becoming a Self-Fulfilling Prophecy

If we choose to, our life can be a self-fulfilling prophecy inspired by the thoughts that inhabit our minds. In all reality, our life is already inspired by these thoughts; if we do not like how our life is being formed right now, we can shift it at any moment.

Undoubtedly, there is no limit to what we can manifest by aligning our minds with the power that has been proven over time. Our capacity for creation, when used intentionally, defies all boundaries and has a timeless efficacy. Through harnessing this power of intention and thought, everything is achievable. As such, star athletes use the power of manifestation to visualize the championship before every competition. Meanwhile, celebrities use the power of affirmations to choose the life they want and the opportunities that come their way.

Using manifestation, we can become our self-fulfilling prophecy. We can prove that others need to believe in their dream life. Yet, if you do not think you will make headway on your goals based on brain research, you are right. But if you shifted your mindset and stepped into positive goal-driven energy, chances are you will amaze yourself. The things you can create simply by thinking about them will be extraordinary. And believe it or not, science has shown that success is sometimes achievable with what we have been led to believe.

For example, you go to bed in a foul mood after a heated exchange with your partner. Disappointed that no resolution was made and angered at the lack of apology from your other half, negative energy fills your being. It is no surprise that this has become a self-fulfilling prophecy as thoughts about the argument keep playing through your head. You cannot help but feel more disgruntled when you spot your partner sound asleep as if nothing had occurred. Hours later, it is time to wake up for work, and you feel like an explosion is imminent. To add fuel to the fire, there is no good morning wish from your partner, only further frustration mounting within you, as if this was not enough trouble already. Likewise, breakfast takes forever while simultaneously getting burned, and your dog decides it is time to relieve itself on the floor. As reality comes crashing down around you, you realize that you neglected laundry last night due to all the quarreling and now have nothing clean to wear, increasing the annoyance towards yourself and maybe even your partner. Your remaining patience is put on thin ice as it resonates in your mind: *"Someone else better not annoys me today!"* So, the universe says, *your wish is my command.*

Feeling overwhelmed and exhausted, you treat yourself to a coffee, only for the barista to get your order wrong. Then, someone even cuts in front of you in line, and an argument ensues. Subsequently, you make it to work only to be laid off by your boss, who informs you that your assistant called in sick. All these feel as if everything was conspiring against you, resulting in the worst day (or week) ever.

Overall, things did not go so well with your partner last night. Despite trying to resolve this, you both went to bed without common ground. That left you feeling worn out, filled with negativity, and completely unappreciative. Breaking all this down can be tough, but you must understand why these feelings arose. This negative behavior shifts the entire trajectory of how your day unfolds. Now, your brain's reticular activating system (RAS) is piqued and alert. We will discuss more how your RAS works in pillar five, so it searches for other ways to fuel your current energy.

In short, the more negative energy you transfer into the universe, the more you receive in your life; it becomes a vast ripple effect of unending negativity unless you wake up one day and decide otherwise.

To manifest a favorable self-fulfilling prophecy, spreading positivity around us is essential. It always begins with three things:

- Your thoughts
- Your behavior
- Your beliefs

Believing in yourself and having an optimistic outlook can lead to a beautiful day. Have faith that you will wake up on time, motivated and beaming with positivity, and the universe will respond to your energy by providing what you desire.

The Law of Attraction is familiar to most of us, but what about the other 11 laws? In the next pillar, we will dive deeper into each one, so you can better understand how to use them for your manifestation goals. With the knowledge of the physics laws that enable manifestation, you will be well on your way to achieving success.

Pillar Two
Laws

Many of us are familiar with the notion that *"like attracts like,"* famously known as the Law of Attraction. This idea is explored in Rhonda Byrne's book *The Secret* and is also referred to in the movie of the same name. *But what about the Law of Polarity? Or the Law of Gender, or even the Law of Vibration?* Together with eight other laws, they make up the Laws of Manifestation, universal principles that align with our spiritual being and allow us to open up an energetic portal for manifestation.

Manifesting our dream life is not only a matter of understanding the Law of Attraction; it is about utilizing all twelve laws. Partnering with the universe is how we can truly become an energetic match for what we desire out of life. Knowing this means understanding how to use each law in its totality, allowing us to manifest our desired reality.

This pillar is about introducing you to the twelve universal laws, which can help us keep pushing forward despite life's challenges. Applying these laws will not magically make your life perfect, but it will bring positivity, abundance, clarity, and contentment.

Understanding them will enable you to live intentionally, compassionately, and with understanding.

Law of Oneness

All living creatures are inextricably linked and part of a common cosmic symphony. Each of these breathing organisms is connected to an abundant energy source that pulses around us. Nothing happens in the universe without us, humans, birds, trees, plants, mammals, flowers, and sea animals, feeling or experiencing it. This connection is like an invisible string that binds us together in one universal force. Think of it like an energetic vibration that unites us all.

Being mindful of our intrinsic link with the world is essential to understand that anything we do, think, and feel affects all of us. When we express negativity to ourselves, it is reflected in our behavior and radiates outwards. Like the people closest to us, our pets are sensitive to this energy. This negativity has far-reaching consequences, eliciting emotions from sadness and frustration to disappointment and anxiety. Interestingly, those surrounding us may also display similar negative vibes, leaving us wondering where they might be coming from. Indeed, since everything is connected at an energetic level, it stands to reason that our energy frequency resonates with that of other living creatures in our environment.

This is the same with happy, uplifting energy. Our positivity and good vibes can be contagious. Those shared moments of joy can help make the world a better place. When we recognize this fundamental idea that we are all connected, it gives us the strength to move forward and use it as our partner on the journey. Gratitude and expression of happiness bring an energy that is both uplifting and inspiring, a feeling of oneness that we should never let go of.

Law of Vibration

The Law of Vibration works in conjunction with the Law of Attraction. Just as the first law states that we are all connected in a universally divine way, it is essential to remember that each of us and non-tangible objects vibrate on a particular vibrational frequency.

When I say non-tangible, I mean items such as desks, ceilings, and the floor, objects that are not living organisms but vibrate on a slower frequency, regardless. As humans, we are always moving and constantly on the go. Therefore, we vibrate at a higher frequency.

To manifest what we want, we need to become an energetic match for them. For example, if you desire to manifest $100,000, you must find a way to become an energetic match for that amount. If you have no idea what that looks like, you can ask yourself these questions:

- What would I be doing?
- How would I present myself?
- How would I make decisions?
- Where would I be hanging out?
- Who would I be hanging out with?
- How would I handle my emotions?

Asking the right questions can bring you closer to your goal of manifesting $100,000. To begin this process, it is essential to identify the way of being and frequency level that larger sums of money operate on. This can be a challenge if you have only been used to working with smaller sums, such as $10,000 or $50,000. So, to match this frequency and truly experience its abundance, you must learn to understand and appreciate it on its unique level. Becoming conscious of what this frequency is capable of will enable you to create the experiences necessary to manifest your desired outcome.

Law of Correspondence

Bre Brown of Modern Manifestation describes the Law of Correspondence as *"what happens around us is a direct reflection of what is happening within us" (2021).* How you feel about yourself reflects how the world perceives and reacts to you. Everything is interconnected, and your inner self directly influences your external environment.

In other words, the reality you are living now is merely a reflection. Maybe you cannot quite understand why you have not achieved as much as you had liked. But it may be due to feelings of scarcity or lack, or self-doubt and fear of failure, which take precedence over any opportunity for success. As such, fear often takes its toll on your prospects, preventing you from taking risks and pushing yourself ahead. This can lead to a cycle of never-ending scarcity and the need to always stay in survival mode. That might be difficult to accept, but do not lose hope; there is still a chance to turn things around.

The more self-aware and candid you can be with yourself, the more successful your journey of growth and change will be. Ergo, replace negative emotions towards your actions or inactions with positive affirmations and show yourself kindness so that what you experience externally reflects how you feel internally. A great way to do this is by practicing the Law of Correspondence. When you believe something good about yourself, that belief manifests into reality. Likewise, find time for self-compassion and understanding as you grow, learn, and progress through life. Granting yourself grace is not easy, but it is crucial in facilitating a healthy inner landscape that will translate positively into our external world.

Law of Attraction

Many people live by the famous law that "like attracts like," and it is all about having a clear mental picture of what you are trying to manifest. For example, if you want a car, you should create a vivid visual of the exact type of car you desire and allow yourself to experience the feeling of owning it. When you take on this mindset, believing that the item is already yours, your energy vibration will match that of owning such an item. Visualizing this in your mind will also help align your thoughts and emotions to attract whatever it is that you wish for actively. As such, focusing on positive thoughts and feelings can help draw things into your life more smoothly.

Meanwhile, radiating negative energy will likely reflect on your life. For the Law of Attraction to work in your favor, practicing positivity and maintaining good mental health is crucial. Refrain from being cruel to yourself, start noticing the good things in your life, and focus on thoughts that make you feel more optimistic about what may come. By eliminating negativity from your mind, you can open yourself up to limitless possibilities; this power should never be underestimated.

The Law of Attraction works like this: Your mental attitude directly affects your life's outcome. When you think positively, creating desirable circumstances is easier. But if you fill yourself with negativity, those same issues will be reflected in the results. Hence, *a positive outlook leads to positive results, while a negative mindset will bring about similarly dismal results.*

Remember the example I shared in pillar one? An argument before bed can leave frustration and annoyance, which will likely still be present when you wake up the following day. Even everyday tasks like making breakfast seem to take forever. Likewise, things like not having clean clothes for work or a barista messing up your coffee order can all be enough to set you off. These minor inconveniences can worsen a bad day and leave a draining feeling; this is an example of a negative ripple effect of pure frustration. Such a case is the opposite of the Law of Attraction. Instead of "like attracts like," it was more like "dislike attracts dislike." Indeed, not a pleasant experience or feeling amidst such a gloomy atmosphere.

But what could happen if you shifted your annoyance and frustration to gratefulness and humility? Chances are, after pushing through the challenge, you and your partner settle into bed feeling grateful for each other. You wake up refreshed, saying good morning to each other with a kiss. Greet your children with enthusiasm, and before long, everyone is ready for breakfast. The two of you enjoy a delicious meal together before getting on with your day and feeling renewed, knowing that you have resolved whatever had been causing friction. You head to the coffee shop and are warmly welcomed by the barista, treating you to a complimentary muffin for being an incredible customer. Upon reaching work, your boss calls you to their office and offers you a promotion that makes you feel elated. Full of cheer and enthusiasm, your assistant asked how your weekend had been while they settled into their daily routine. All these were a great start to the day.

See the difference between feeling frustrated the night before to feeling energetic, motivated, and optimistic? The Law of Attraction is a matter of simple perception. Desiring to manifest extraordinary things requires your feelings and thoughts to hold the same positive energy.

Law of Action

By taking inspired action, you can manifest your dreams and bring yourself closer to the things you want. It is a powerful tool that works hand-in-hand with the Law of Attraction. When approached positively, these two forces can produce beautiful results. However, it is important to note that they will only do something if you take action. For instance, while simply dreaming of a far-off destination is excellent, it will only amount to a little once you start taking steps toward making it happen. This could involve writing down why it is your dream vacation spot and adding it to your vision board or researching the area and budgeting for the trip. Taking action in an inspired way will help bring your vision into reality quicker than just thinking about it alone. *Yet, the Law of Action is not about taking the right action; it is about choosing to take a step, no matter what.* To be frank, we have no idea what can happen when we take action, but we know that we are taking the next step, and the outcome will be revealed to us when it is time.

Despite that, people fearing the unknown paralyze and keep them from achieving their goals. To combat this, we must take action, no matter the outcome. While it might not always lead to the desired result, it still teaches valuable lessons about perseverance and resilience. Taking small steps towards our goal can also help build courage and push past our fears. Aside from that, learning we may fail should not stop us from trying since any experience gained will benefit us in the long run. And if we successfully take action, we reap the rewards of our efforts and get closer to achieving our manifested desires. Likewise, in finding out what lies ahead, we must take the first step regardless of how scary or uncertain it may seem. Either way, it is a win-win and meant for celebration.

Alongside that, many people wrongly assume that using the Law of Attraction is enough to receive their desired outcome without effort. It appears too good to be true; if it were, as such, everybody in the world would have their wishes come true while they sit on the couch watching TV. However, this is not the case. The power of manifestation is realized when we combine positive affirmations with taking action toward our goals. When we take the time to understand this concept better, our dreams can manifest at just the right times. By combining visualization techniques with hard work and dedication, we can achieve our goals more quickly. This process can help us foster meaningful growth and transformation in our lives— something that could otherwise not be accomplished by sitting idle and hoping for something to happen.

Law of Perpetual Transmutation of Energy

By surrounding ourselves with positive energy, internally and externally, we can create a flow of uplifting emotion that radiates out into the world. This idea of positivity in motion has profound implications: when we let go of negative thinking, our internal state shifts in a way that resonates throughout the universe. On the other hand, if we focus on gratitude and happiness, these positive vibrations spread outwards and bring balance to our environment. As you intentionally cultivate an attitude of contentment and joy, you can manifest positive energy that reverberates in both personal and communal life.

For instance, the consequences are usually dire if you stay in negative energy. Likely, you may experience job loss, anxiety, unhealthy relationships, and an overall feeling that life is bleak. Subsequently, you can become overwhelmed with bills and have more bad days than good. But recognizing your negativity and taking steps to counter it through practicing gratitude can rewire your thought patterns and attract more positive experiences. Focusing on the good things in life can make joy, opportunity, contentment, and security you put forth the effort to shift your mindset away from negative thinking.

Replacing negative energy with positive and abundant feelings can be transformational. You can manifest the relationships, experiences, and resources you desire, such as a fulfilling partnership, an exciting vacation, loving friendships that offer encouragement and support, and financial security. These possibilities create a radically different atmosphere than one filled with negativity. Then, instead of fear or worry, you will experience joy, excitement, gratitude, and contentment.

Clearly, this law is about how we choose to transmute our internal energy. Learning to manifest constant positive energy can lead to a few things:

- Surrounding yourself with positive people that become your circle of influence. When you surround yourself

with positive energy, your internal energy will translate into the same.
- Having better-feeling thoughts. Be kind to yourself and show self-compassion every day. Treat yourself with the love and respect you deserve so it flows back to you.
- Becoming a constant co-creator with the universe. The universe usually gives you what you want when you ask for it. Perhaps it is not in the moment, but as long as you are taking inspired action toward your goals, the universe will help make things happen.
- Constantly feeling abundant and grateful. As long as you already think abundant, despite what you do not have, the universe will conspire with you to give you more while helping you release attachment to the outcome. Feel grateful for what you have now, as gratefulness aligns with positive energy, which helps bring more abundance your way.

All these things can help transmute your energy into abundance and positivity. When your energy exhibits a flow of this caliber, you will notice that it feels easier to manifest exactly what you want rather than manifest negatively because you are transmuting negative energy within you.

With anything you learn about manifestation in this book, understand that the way you transmute your energy into the world is the way that you will manifest. Knowing this, you will find a way to shift your energy from negative to positive, so your life can drastically change for the better.

Law of Cause and Effect

Newton says, *"For every action, there is an equal and opposite reaction."* Every action you take has a certain effect on your life. This feels pretty straightforward, but in reality, many of us forget how this law can play into our lives. Nothing can really happen if we do not take a single action in our life. *Pretty simple, right?* Due to this, we cannot realistically expect to manifest what we want if we do not take a single step toward our goals.

When you entertain a scarcity mindset, it can hurt your life. This could manifest itself through feelings of lack, stress, anxiety, or worry. It is worth noting that by not doing anything to strive for your desired outcome, you still took action. Because it will still give you a result. It might not be the results you wanted, but results, nonetheless. The Law of Cause and Effect emphasizes how our choices and behaviors in the present shape our future circumstances. That's why having a proactive attitude is essential if you want financial freedom and abundance.

Once you become aware of this, the best thing to do is make the shift. Instead of getting anxious over a possible future and clouding your mind with stress and pessimism, practice positive thinking and take action for what you truly want to create. This will help you craft the life of your dreams from the steps you take based on those inspired decisions. The results of these decisions become a vast ripple effect portrayed in our lives. Many of us believe that nothing good comes from our actions, but I choose to have a different outlook. Even if things did not work out the way I expected, I still feel grateful for the lessons I have learned throughout the journey. I have taken the actions I was guided to take; therefore, the results become an energetic match and will continue aligning in the way they are meant to be.

Every action we take or do not take has a consequence; this is the belief of this law. Negative actions, such as lacking gratitude or waiting for things to come to you, will result in unfavorable reactions. As such, we would not get what we want, experience constant scarcity, or feel a lack. *So, how can you use this law to your advantage and achieve extraordinary effects?* To do this, you must understand that every action has an equal reaction and be conscious of your behavior to ensure the desired outcomes. Likewise, you must—

- Understand why you are taking the actions. If it feels inspiring, you will move forward with it and experience beautiful results because of it.
- Embrace everything, both pleasant and unpleasant; make peace with all that shapes your life's path, and appreciate every single part.
- Be clear on the results you want to achieve. When you have clarity, you will know what actions to take so the results can manifest.
- Trust yourself and the universe. The results may not be what you expected them to be, but eventually, you will understand that they are so much better.
- Surrender to what is meant to be. Release complete attachment to the outcome. Know and believe that your actions are more than enough to manifest what you desire and allow the universe to do its thing.

In short, to spark change and transformation, take the inspired actions required to invoke that change.

Law of Compensation

Have you ever heard the saying, *"what goes around comes around"*? The Law of Compensation is a universal principle that aligns with this notion: *whatever energy and actions you put into the world will be repaid with the same.* Be mindful of this when considering your actions and how they may come back to you; think positive, positive returns. When you dwell on negative actions and attitudes, it will cast a shadow on your life. As the saying goes, "Karma will get you." On the contrary, when you exude positive energy, you can expect to be rewarded for your efforts. Remember, it is all about sowing good seeds.

Helping and serving others can be rewarding, but you may find that the universe pays you back. The Law of Compensation is linked to your perceptions; taking positive steps toward fulfilling your dreams will bring back the same energy from the universe. Likewise, this law relates to your mentality. Keeping an outlook of lack or insecurity will only lead to more instances that confirm those feelings. On the contrary, having a mindset of abundance and self-love will draw forth more love and a wellspring into your life.

The actions you take determine how you are compensated. If you are ungrateful for the things you currently have, chances are you will not receive more for a while. But if you are eternally grateful for all that you have, you will receive more things to be grateful for. *See how this works?* When you think about it, it is instead a simple concept. Bottom line, *say thank you for all that you have, and the universe will say, "you are welcome."*

As Wayne Dyer famously quoted, *"When you change the way you look at things, the things you look at change."* This simple phrase exemplifies the Law of Compensation; an example demonstrated daily. If we take a moment to reframe our perspective, the objects we observe will likewise be altered. So, when you are facing hard times, finding ways to shift your outlook in your mind and reality is essential. Yet, focusing on the struggles and all the intense emotions that come with them, such as fear, stress, anxiety, disappointment, or worry, you will notice that same energy in the physical world. Perhaps, it is terrible news taking over your social media feeds, family appearing grumpy more often, or a sense of self-loathing; each can become an obstacle when attempting to tackle challenging situations and only make things worse. Somehow it feels like all these negative feelings have skyrocketed overnight, and you wonder if there is ever an end in sight. However, there is hope if you work on controlling your mindset and finding the light at the end of the tunnel.

Clearly, a reminder of The Law of Compensation is that at any moment, you have the power to change your mindset. Every 24 hours allows us to go about our day with positive actions and attitudes. However, if we do not do this and would instead view things from a pessimistic viewpoint, it is entirely up to us.

The Law of Relativity

The Law of Relativity, also referred to as the Law of Perspective, explains how everything is relative. As such, everything in your life is always happening, so you can learn, grow, and celebrate. Yet, it also greatly depends on your perspective of why things are happening. Depending on the way you perceive the situation, it can lead to either success or failure. For example, we can go through a traumatic breakup, and our minds can have two different perspectives:

1. *Why do bad things always happen to me? Why do I always attract the wrong people? What is wrong with me? Am I not lovable?* Or;
2. *What can I learn from this breakup so it does not happen again? How has it made me stronger? More confident? Resilient?*

Perspective can make a world of difference in our outlook on life. We have the choice to either remain emotionally distant, believing that we are undeserving of good fortune and abundance, or to look ahead toward the potential for self-improvement. When faced with certain situations, these experiences have likely been granted to us so that we can understand them and become more resilient if they arise again. As we progress, our journey may lead us toward becoming a better version of ourselves.

On the Law of Relativity, our perspective means more to us and our manifestations than we may realize. Suppose you desire to manifest your dream vehicle, and it does not show up when you expected it to. In that case, you can either believe that manifestation does not work and you will never get the car, or you can assume that your dream car will show up when it is meant to. Until then, you must be grateful for the car you have now and keep taking inspired action until it arrives, regardless of how long it takes.

Notice the difference in energy?

Half the population will offer a negative perspective on the situations they experience. Meanwhile, the other half will think positively and still believe that everything is possible and that there is pure potential in the world. Think about the *"glass empty or full" analogy. What do you believe? Is the glass half full? Or is it half empty?* Your perspective of this analogy will determine how the Law of Relativity shows up in your life.

Law of Polarity

The Law of Polarity is about understanding that everything in life comes in pairs. Negativity versus positivity, light versus darkness, white versus black, healthy versus sick, self-doubt versus confidence—everything that makes us both human and spirit has an opposite partner attached to it. When we understand this perspective, we know how to shift our minds, attitude, and behavior to see the brighter side of the not-so-great experiences we may witness, and then we have something to look forward to.

Life is full of duality; we understand this well. Consider when you are launching a business, and suddenly something happens, like a family member getting sick or your partner asking for a divorce. You can either feel like the world is ending and question whether you should pursue it or take it in stride and trust that you will learn valuable lessons about resilience, strength, and personal growth. These moments give us chances to learn how best to handle our lives no matter how difficult they become.

Some may believe they are being punished because they want to do something good, but the universe is not around for punishment. One thing remains true no matter how dark it gets; light always finds a way. This is the Law of Polarity, reminding us that no matter what happens, there is an undeniable balance in our lives. Just as we can hold the goodness that shows up in our lives, we also have the strength and the money to move through the darkness when faced with a challenge. According to the Law of Polarity, we can gain valuable insight and knowledge from our experiences while still being able to choose how we view them. Through each choice, we can make the most out of any situation and grow in different ways.

Law of Rhythm

As the seasons transition, so can you. Being mindful of the Law of Rhythm is essential for realizing your desires; all that is required is to move through life's peaks and valleys and accept what fate has in store for you. It means letting go of what you can't control and embracing those that you're unable to change.

There are a few things to remember when focusing on this law:

- Let go of the past. Feeling stuck, never moving forward, does not allow you to move in the rhythmic flow of life.
- Enjoy life exactly how the experiences are meant to play out in your life. They may not be the greatest experiences, but they are moments of lessons and growth. Trust them.
- Release negativity and find ways to move forward positively.
- Let go of the person you once were, so you can flow and align yourself with the person you are meant to become—your next-level self.

Have you ever wanted something extraordinary, like a dream job or more money in your bank account, yet it never comes to be? It could be because you are not allowing yourself to move forward abundantly. Likely, you may stop wealth and prosperity from coming your way due to limiting beliefs, and negative emotions held deep within you. Ask yourself, *"are these obstacles holding me back?"* Reflect on these a bit and see how you can make changes to live abundantly. By releasing all the negative energy, you open yourself up to more flow and a positive rhythm that helps open doors to a greater life.

Law of Gender

This law is about achieving harmony and manifesting our goals without struggle. Do not be misled by its name; it has nothing to do with gender or sex. By creating an equilibrium between masculine and feminine energy, we can find joy, peace, and tranquility. Achieving balance is the secret to unlocking a life of happiness and contentment.

For those new to understanding masculine and feminine energy, here is a simple breakdown between the two. Masculine energy is about actions making your dreams come true. Taking those bold steps, strategizing, formulating a plan of action, and setting goals all require the work of this powerful energy in your life. Through these inspired actions, you can reach the heights you have been aiming for. Meanwhile, feminine energy is a journey of trusting your emotions and embracing life. Knowing how achieving your goals will make you feel will help guide your decisions. Believe that all the things you wish for are already yours, even if they have yet to appear. Allow yourself to be open and receive them when it is time.

In human experience, you cannot have one without the other. You can embrace more masculine energy than feminine energy and vice versa. Yet, you live your life daily with both energies within you. Understanding this concept lets you know how the Law of Gender can work in your life. By creating a beautiful harmonious balance between both energies, the Law of Gender works in your life and aligns your actions so your manifestations can come to fruition.

After breaking down the meaning behind all 12 manifestation laws, comprehend how to apply them to elevate your energetic vibration. When those vibrations match up to the same level as your manifestations, it is a natural occurrence. Learning about the third pillar can be incredibly helpful in grasping and raising that vibration for a more abundant life.

Pillar Three
Vibration

Each one of us has an energetic vibration within us. As humans, we are made up of millions of cells, and these cells produce a wave of vibrational energy. Our world is filled with a constantly buzzing energy. Hear it in your heartbeat and the wind, feel it as your feet touch the ground when you walk, and sense it with every nerve ending in your body. From the unseen rhythms to what you can see, we are surrounded by vibration, an energy that pulsates through us all.

By understanding how vibrational energy works within us, we can manifest our desired abundance, love, health, and spirituality. This chapter will provide an overview of the connection between thoughts, behaviors, and vibrations that flow at the highest frequency for manifestation. Furthermore, we will discuss strategies to elevate our energetic vibration, such as thanksgiving, breathwork practices, meditation, and energy therapy. Knowing the power of our vibrational energy is crucial to achieving a life full of joy.

What Is Vibrational Energy?

Some have described vibrational energy as a *"box of emotions"* *(Goswami, 2021)*. Experiencing low vibrational energy leads to fear, grief, sadness, worry, stress, and disappointment. Conversely, raising your vibration allows you to recognize the feelings of happiness, peace, joy, abundance, compassion, and unconditional love. By tuning into these emotions more regularly, you can create a happier life with greater contentment.

When manifesting, vibrational energy is about tuning into a positive, energetic frequency that makes you feel excited and grateful to tap into the energy of what you want. Experiencing vibrational energy is like connecting to the Laws of Rhythm, Vibration, and Attraction. Our desire moves us; what we want to do drives our actions. We act out of choice, not necessity. Stepping into a higher vibrational frequency is as if we are choosing to turn up the music so we can no longer hear the white noise in the background that distracts us from achieving our goals. The white noise, also known as negative vibrational energy, could be limiting beliefs, negative self-talk, worry, fear, self-doubt, imposter syndrome, anxiety, lack of self-trust and confidence, and trying to do everything all on our own.

As we all know, our energetic vibration is composed mostly of pure energy, so we must be aware of how we feel. To gauge your energy at the moment, look at what you are listening to on the radio. Hearing dark and heavy tunes that have an isolating effect could signal that something is not right emotionally. Or if you are more drawn to upbeat and optimistic songs with positive messages, it could mean you are in a celebration mode and feeling good about life. Reflect on the emotions that determine your current vibrational energy; if it is not quite where you want it to be, do not hesitate to redirect.

What Are Vibrational Beings?

Vibrational beings are not any one thing; it is all of us. Our vibrational frequency is a state of being; it is how we live. As we have stated previously, we can be a high vibrational being or operate as a low vibrational being. This depends on how we react to certain situations or experiences and the emotions that drive our reactions to those experiences.

There will be moments in our life when we may feel anxious, stressed, worried, self-doubt, or even at the worst extreme, depressed. In these moments, we are operating as a low vibrational being. We feel lost, perhaps overworked and underappreciated; therefore, our state of being is negative. Remaining in this vibration can be a deterrent that will steer us in the opposite direction of our dreams, as it can create a downward spiral of negative emotions. Without a second thought, we slip into a dark abyss, our minds soon entangled by depression. Before we know it, the feeling has deeply rooted itself within us.

When it comes to manifesting, being in a state of positivity, abundance, and gratitude is essential. Focusing on creating an uplifted, inspired, and empowered mindset is vital for our manifestations to come true. We need to be aware of the frequency we are currently vibrating at and work towards shifting it into one that resonates with these positive energies. Doing this daily can create instantaneous changes in our vibration and make our desires tangible.

Connection of Thoughts, Behaviors, and Vibrations

*"You do not manifest what you want;
you attract what you are."*
–Francesco Filippazzo

Connecting with ourselves is simple. Having negative thoughts brings us down to low vibration. This low energy affects our behavior; before we know it, we have manifested what we did not want instead of what we did.

For instance, negative thoughts start to creep in when we lack self-confidence. We tell ourselves our goals will not be achieved and that we do not have the knowledge or experience to succeed. This leads to procrastination, feeling like an imposter, lacking action, and being unmotivated. As such, when potential clients turn down our services, it compounds these feelings of inadequacy, leading us to become less creative and less motivated toward achieving our dreams. Eventually, we may even start doubting the power of manifestation or the Law of Attraction. All of these result from low vibrational frequency; before long, we begin losing sight of our visions and dreams, forgetting who we are, and going through an identity crisis. From that, we can quickly become convinced that failure is inevitable and feeling unhappy is all we deserve.

This is an overreaching example of low vibrational energy, but you can see how deep the connection can be to our behavior, actions, and thoughts. There is a science to this, which I will explain in the following sections so you can gather a deeper understanding of our connection to the universe and ourselves.

The Science of Vibration

Vibrational frequency is a phenomenon for many people. Like other things regarding energetics—affirmations, manifestation, Law of Attraction, spirituality, and God—many people believe that it must not be accurate if you cannot see them physically. Yet, some people struggle to believe in things they cannot see with their own eyes, leading to cynicism about the world around them. This kind of thinking leads to a mistrustful worldview and gives birth to misanthropes.

However, if you were to look at this from a scientific perspective, we know that gravity exists, even if we cannot see it. *How would humans keep their feet on the ground when walking? How would we go headfirst toward the ground if we were to jump off a building? How would astronauts float in the air when they are in space without gravity holding them down?* Gravity is not a tangible product; it is a force of nature that is proven by our actions and behaviors. We cannot physically see gravity, yet, it exists.

This same belief can be brought forth when speaking about vibrational frequency. Though we cannot physically see them, vibrations have a powerful hold over us, especially when it comes to music. We groove to the rhythm of the tunes at parties and feel our favorite songs reverberate within us whenever they come on the radio. There is no denying that the energy of music captivates us completely. As we are connected to different energy sources by a certain vibrational frequency, we can be sure that our manifestations will come to fruition depending on the wavelength we are vibrating on.

Unfortunately, people often think it is not real if they do not see proof of manifestation coming true quickly. We tend to doubt the universe when our desired outcomes do not happen as expected, for example, expecting $10,000 to show up in your account by next month and concluding that manifestation does not work if it does not come through. However, this kind of thinking needs to be revised; evidence of a manifestation can be seen later for us to believe in its power. Even if what we want is not brought into our lives instantly, that is still no indication that it can never exist.

When it comes to vibration, it may seem odd at first glance. However, take electricity as an example; it is a natural force that has been around for thousands and years and is found everywhere around the globe *(Wonderopolis, 2019)*. Similarly to the idea of manifestation and gravity, although it cannot be seen with our eyes, it still counts as an absolute concept. Evidence for its realness is all around us; when we turn on our TVs, plug in our laptops to charge them, or put on our morning blender, we realize it is true. The proof that electricity exists lies within us and in science and spirituality, no matter how much we may not be able to witness its effects with sight.

In other words, we cannot physically see the vibration, but that does not mean it does not exist. Vibration is just like electricity. We cannot physically see electricity, but we can feel its energy anytime we do our daily activities. Many things we cannot see with our naked eye are incomprehensible; that is the beauty of science. All of our dreams exist on a specific vibrational frequency. As our current selves, we may not vibrate on the same level as our dreams, but that does not mean our dreams are not meant for us. Taking inspired action every day is vital to achieving our goals. When we put in the effort towards inner growth, we find ourselves resonating at a higher frequency, enabling us to bring our aspirations into physical reality.

Positive and High-frequency Vibration

To better comprehend positive and negative vibrations, start by exploring the science behind vibrational energy. This understanding will allow you to become aware of your vibration levels. In cases when it is on a negative scale, you will know what actions to take to bring it back up.

Positive manifestation operates on a high-level frequency. Many emotions are associated with this level, such as happiness, joy, peace, abundance, gratitude, acceptance, love, and courage. As you feel authentically happy, more things to feel satisfied with flow to you. When you feel peaceful, you become aware and mindful of experiences around you that help instill calm and greater harmony. In short, the more you feel grateful for what you currently have, the more the universe will give you to be grateful for.

For instance, let us say you are striving to make your dream career a reality. Feeling ecstatic and ready for the world, you purchase an outfit that will give you a professional edge in interviews. Likewise, you affirm that this dream job is on its way to you, but weeks go by, and you are still waiting for a response from potential employers. Anxiety and stress may creep in, but it is okay. Remind yourself that your ideal job will come when it is meant to happen, then shift your mindset to be positive again. Send out resumes and create connections with companies while appreciating what your current job has given you, even if it is not the role of your dreams yet. Then, one day, as if by magic, you receive a call from the employer who has captivated your attention. Regardless of its outcome, remain excited and optimistic with gratitude. This chance is to show them your enthusiasm and passion first-hand. As your energy reverberates, they offer you the job.

This example shows that you draw in what reflects your thoughts. If you are sitting around, being cynical about achieving your goals, you might find yourself in a detrimental cycle, likely to bring negative happenings. Conversely, if you take time to motivate and equip yourself and act on impetus towards attaining your objectives, you will be back on track to draw in the outcomes of your desires at a faster rate.

Hence, high-frequency vibration is a science in its own right. What you are today determines what you will attract. If your feelings and emotions are consistently balanced, optimistic, and serene, this will bring more peace, bliss, and joy into your life. However, it can be hard to remain in a positive state all the time. As human beings, we must acknowledge that moments of hardship or despair might come our way but do not have to be discouraging. When we become aware of our mental, physical, and spiritual selves, we can regain the power to transform these moments into more empowering and high-frequency vibrations.

Negative and Low-frequency Vibration

Negative vibration works like this: *The more you think, act, and behave negatively, the more negative experiences you attract into your life.* Low-frequency emotions include stress, worry, fear, anxiety, guilt, shame, pride, grief, and anger. When you feel any of these emotions, you enter a negative energetic frequency that can stop you from receiving what you want. Becoming aware of your feelings is a must to change the energy you are giving off. Taking time to be mindful of our emotions helps us shift into a positive vibe that will attract the things we desire, not what we do not. By recognizing and reorganizing our thoughts, we can move in alignment with manifesting the abundance we long for.

As such, let us assume that you want to manifest the relationship of your dreams. That said, you will need to shift away from the energetic vibrations from past harmful connections. Here is an example; say your desire is for a supportive partner. All too often, your history has been built on toxicity and destruction. Now, they have created an unconscious belief that you are not good enough or worthy of having the relationship you want. Instead of love, resentment lingers; instead of self-acceptance, a sense of unworthiness and lack of appreciation abounds. Gratitude is replaced by feeling undeserving of unconditional love, while feelings of scarcity and lack substitute abundance. All these emotions keep you firmly in the depths of low energy. And when you feel stuck in low energy, you go down a dark rabbit hole of deeper negative emotions, such as anger, doubt, worry, stress, hatred, rejection, and pride.

Fostering these negative emotions can be detrimental, leading to an increased risk of attracting people and situations with the same low vibes, which can cause further damage than you are conscious of. Acknowledging these emotions is essential, as no good will come from them aside from self-awareness and the chance to shift into a better state. Some common signs that you are stuck in a negative spiral are constantly doubting yourself, picking on yourself negatively, speaking badly about others, and continually feeling angry. Recognizing this allows you to work on improving your mental state.

Observation and Self-Awareness

Our day-to-day behavior and habits often become so entrenched that we do not notice how they affect our self-image and how we present ourselves to others. Breaking out of this cycle of negative thoughts and limited beliefs is challenging, but it is possible with a little conscious effort. Practicing self-awareness can help us to identify when unhelpful behavior patterns emerge, allowing us to make the changes necessary to alter those patterns for the better. It takes time and patience, but by being mindful of our actions, we can eventually overcome our default thought processes and develop healthier ones. With enough practice and commitment, these new behaviors will soon become second nature, helping us live more fulfilling lives where we are more at ease with ourselves.

Unfortunately, many people have spent most of their lifetime belittling themselves and embracing their limiting beliefs. These are the same people who want to change their lives and transform their mindset, but they do not know how, so they continue to run around on the hamster wheel of life, never moving forward. Yet, to make a difference, one can start taking the time to observe and practice self-awareness. As such, slow your conversations when speaking with others so you can notice the words you use. Intentionally pay attention to the way you talk to yourself by bringing these words to your conscious state of mind. Then, if your loved one is in a lousy mood, compliment them. Counteract their behavior with positive sentiments. Tell them you love them, how grateful you are for their presence in your life, and what you love about them. Surely, you will notice a shift in their energy immediately. On the other hand, the worst thing you can do in this situation is to join them in their negative energy.

In pillar six, we will go into further detail, but the bottom line is that your words can enhance or diminish somebody's life and your own. Ergo, your speech has the power to alter your destiny. Remember this as you speak to someone and yourself. Since this power is within you, it can instantly raise your vibration and others. By becoming aware and observing your energy and the energy of those around you, you can transform your mindset and others, making your environment an empowering place to be in.

Raising Your Vibration

Now that you have a deeper understanding of the differences between positive and negative vibration, there are many ways that you can implement this right away that will help you raise your vibration. Manifesting positively is about three essential things: *taking inspired action, being intentional with who you are and where you are currently, and feeling grateful for what you have.* Here are some ways to raise your vibration to a higher energetic frequency for a more abundant life.

Love

Love is amongst the highest forms of energetic vibration. Simply put, if you want to raise your vibration immediately, express love to others and yourself. Tell your loved ones how much you love them, express compassion and care for those in need, look in the mirror daily, and tell yourself how much you love and appreciate yourself.

Aside from that, you can also think of the people you love and how they bring joy to your life. A unique way of meditating and visualizing them can raise your vibration instantly. Relax in a quiet area, free from distractions. Recall their smile, laughter, and conversations with you; what they do makes you feel warm inside. Remember the last talk you had and activities like making dinner for you, calling to say hi, or even bringing chicken soup when work or illness drained your energy. Performing this exercise frequently will lift your energetic vibration quickly.

Showing affection is a simple act that can make immense changes in your life and those around you. *The more love you share, the higher your energy vibration is, and the more your outlook shifts.*

Forgiveness

To raise your vibration, forgiveness is an important one. When you are in a negative state of mind, feelings of guilt, shame, anger, annoyance, and frustration toward yourself and those around you can cause your energetic frequency to plummet. Likewise, this will only attract more negativity into your life. Although it may feel difficult, you must learn to forgive, not just for your well-being but for the well-being of others.

Of course, forgiveness does not happen overnight, as it takes time to process, analyze, and heal. Yet, writing a letter to yourself and others is proven effective when learning to forgive. You do not have to give it to the person if you choose not to; however, writing your thoughts and how you feel toward the situation rather than keeping them bottled up inside has been proven to help you effectively heal. Suppose you are in the process of forgiving yourself. In that case, you can also write a forgiveness letter to yourself apologizing for being a self-inflicted bully and beating you up instead of offering unconditional love and support. Through the process of forgiveness, you can release all the negative weight and excess baggage that is weighing you down, which in turn, makes room for positive and empowering energy.

Use Your Five Senses

Raising your vibration is about focusing on positive energy in and around you. There is abundance everywhere you look. Feeling abundant is one of the highest forms of positive energy. Learning to use all five senses will help you notice every area of abundance in your life.

- **Smell:** Take notice of the things that smell beautiful around you. The flowers, trees, coffee brewing in the morning, preparing your meals, having a glass of wine, the scent of a baby's skin, your bubble bath, the shampoo and conditioner as you lather your hair in the shower, your partner's cologne, how you smell after you first get out of the shower, the lotion you lather your body with—your nose is engulfed with scents every day. For a fun, sweet-smelling surprise, you can also walk to your favorite bakery or bake some cookies and take in how delicious they smell. Noticing simple things about our everyday life and breathing them in can help raise your vibration and experience gratitude.
- **See:** Acknowledge all the beauty around you. The way your partner smiles at you, the way they look at you, the infinite beauty of the flowers and other parts of nature, when the snow falls on the ground and glistens in the moonlight, watching a romantic movie with your loved ones, witnessing the beauty of the sunrise or sunset, reading inspiring words to start your day, reading your favorite book, the looks

on your family's faces when you bring dinner to the table, their expressions when the meal is delicious—there is so much beauty around us that we can view with our naked eye.

- **Hear:** Beautiful sounds can raise our energy. Hearing your partner's voice on the phone when they call you simply because they are thinking of you, listening to your favorite song or band, hearing your dog bark when they are happy to see you, listening to an empowering podcast about personal growth, your children's laughter, the sound of a payment notification, the unexpected call from a friend you have not heard from in a long time, a high energy song on the radio.
- **Taste:** Experiencing the kiss of your special someone, having a spoonful of your favorite ice cream or dessert, savoring a delicious home-cooked meal made by your partner, sipping on an exquisite glass of wine or cocktail, or even just taking a gulp of refreshing water—all these can excite and tantalize your taste buds. When this happens, you feel as if an energetic spark has been ignited within you.
- **Feel:** From the smoothness of your partner's skin to petting your cat when you return home, take a moment to notice the feel-good moments that happen in daily life. The loofah gliding over your body in the shower, the hot water and bubbles in a bath, and the musical rhythm as you dance to your favorite songs are all reasons to express love and gratitude. Feel the warmth of hugs from your kids every night before bed, or try gripping hands with your loved

one if it has been a while since you have seen them. Do not forget how amazing it feels when someone compliments you or how great it is to make someone else feel special. Finally, take pride in completing projects, or rejoice in celebratory moments. By simply being aware of these positives around you and how they make you feel, your vibration at that moment can be raised exponentially.

Breathwork

The pace of our lives can often be overwhelming, leading to stress and anxiety. Practices like breathwork offer us a chance to find solace in the present and break away from the hustle and bustle. We often become so preoccupied with everyday tasks that we forget to prioritize living in the here and now and focus on surviving. Breathwork is a great way to pause, take a deep breath, and re-focus on the present, a guide for peace and tranquility.

Deep breathing helps you focus more on what truly matters: finding peace. Peace is a high vibe feeling. When you feel constant peace, despite what is happening around you, you vibrate at a higher frequency, allowing you to manifest more easily. There are many benefits to breathwork:

- Feeling calm
- Mindfulness
- Increases positivity
- Sense of peace
- Releases stress and anxiety
- Sense of joy and fulfillment
- Improves bodily functions, such as the heart and lungs

Meditation

Meditating is another excellent way of focusing on the present moment. It allows you to focus on the present and instills peace, joy, fulfillment, and a sense of purpose. Likewise, it helps remind you that you have a purpose on this planet and offers you abundance and prosperity. Combining breathwork while meditating is also great, as it allows you to focus more intentionally on how your body feels. Lastly, through meditation, you can dive into your emotions and understand how you are feeling.

Under pressure, meditation is a great way to alleviate this feeling and focus on finding inner peace if you are feeling anxious. Regular practice can help you identify where this anxiety stems from so you can be freed from it. Besides, meditating only takes a few minutes to raise your vibration and reap its long-term benefits. However, consistency is critical to fully experiencing these effects.

There are many ways to meditate. Some of the common ways are listed below:

- **Sitting with your legs crossed, eyes closed, and palms facing up in a receiving position.** Going for a guided meditation can be an enjoyable experience, or you may opt for the quiet practice of paying attention to your internal sensations and environmental noises. This silent meditation can help center your energy, allowing you to achieve higher vibrations without distractions. Focus solely on yourself and your surroundings and remember to note any changes.

- **Laying down on your back in a comfortable position.** Close your eyes and take a few moments to immerse yourself in the calming experience of your favorite meditation music. Let the soundwaves wash over you and drift away on a journey of relaxation. Allow yourself to relax as the music envelops you completely. On the other hand, you can choose to focus on your breathwork. Forget about anything happening around you and focus on deep breathing to find a sense of calm and peace.
- **With crystals and chakras.** Placing crystals on your heart, sacral, or solar plexus chakras can raise high vibrational energy. Clear quartz, rose quartz, citrine, and amethyst are perfect for this purpose. Intend to focus intensely while taking slow and steady breaths; you will soon feel the positive effects of crystal energy.

Gratitude

> "You cannot feel fear or anger while feeling gratitude at the same time."
> *–Tony Robbins*

Appreciating all you have in life puts out a positive energy and karma that rewards you in return. Expressing gratitude for what you possess today brings more to be thankful for in the future. Hence, being grateful for your current state is essential for achieving higher levels of joy.

To put gratitude into motion, here are a couple of exercises you can participate in.

- **Start a gratitude journal.** In being grateful, small things can be just as important as the big ones. Challenge yourself to come up with five things to be thankful for. It may seem easy, but it is surprisingly difficult for many people. For example, you could express gratitude for that morning cup of coffee made by your partner or the sun streaming in through your window and waking you up with its warm glow. But even if those things do not feel like much, they are worth reflecting on and appreciating. So, take time to focus on what makes you happy, no matter how insignificant it may seem.
- **Seize a moment to look around you and notice everything you are surrounded by.** Breathe them in and feel grateful for them. Take notice of them. Recognize the everyday wonders in life. Appreciate how amazing it is to have a partner that loves you, your children's joyous laughter, and the sheer delight of being welcomed by your pup each day. Cherish the sustenance that nourishes you—food and water. Show gratitude to those around you, like your neighbor who clears the path for you and the air that carries us all on its gentle breeze. Acknowledge each morning for letting you open your eyes to another opportunity in life. Overall, gratitude is a simple yet powerful emotion we often take for granted when fear, stress, and anxiety overtake us. Likewise, to get into a higher vibrational state of consciousness, feel grateful for who you are and what you have now.

Generosity

To lift your energetic frequency, look for ways to be more generous. Refrain from giving away all your resources but find ways to support those in need. Draw in the same energy you are radiating; if you desire financial prosperity and fertility, consider offering some of this abundance. Similarly, if you hope for a beautiful connection with a partner, focus on building positive relationships with the individuals around you.

In terms of vibrational frequency, compassion and generosity are higher. Meanwhile, scarcity and lack are not; therefore, you stay on the low vibration scale if you feel stingy with your money and your help. But if you do all that you can to offer your support and service to those around you, you feel generous, and it makes you feel good, instilling positivity in your spirit. Positivity leads to good fortune.

Diet

Eating food and consuming drinks that give you a lot of energy is essential. By creating a well-balanced diet, you consume more energy-rich food than food that does not offer you the nutrients and energy you need, such as junk food, sugar-based food, or food that contains high amounts of carbohydrates or sodium. Food such as these keeps you in a low vibrational state and produces fatigue, anxiety, bloatedness, and sleep deprivation, which can make you feel sick, lack focus and motivation, and increase stress. Hence, *the more natural, the better.*

Food and drinks that are high in energy include:

- Organic fruit and veggies (not frozen peas, strawberries, or other fruits and veggies that come from your freezer)
- Avocados
- Food that is high in protein, such as eggs and fish
- Beans and legumes

- Nuts
- Water
- Organic and natural fruit juices
- Green drinks and smoothies
- Teas

Energy Therapy

Energy therapy has proven to be effective for many, many years. These techniques combine spiritual forces of energy in and around you in order to create a hormonal balance that promotes health and well-being. There are times that we feel stuck and confused, and it seems like we are doing everything right, but our internal energy still feels off. Participating in the form of energy therapy can help balance our energy and alleviate any internal blockages that are getting in the way.

There are various types of energy therapy that you can participate in that will greatly help in raising your vibration:

- **Reiki:** With reiki, we can learn to harness our own inner strength and start the process of recovery. Through scientific research, scientists have proven that we have the power within us to heal ourselves; reiki is performed using the foundation of this belief. A professionally trained practitioner can use universal powers combined with the client's energetic frequency to help promote the body's natural ability to heal. Many people diagnosed with cancer and other illnesses have undergone reiki therapy sessions and seen positive effects.
- **Acupuncture:** Drawing from the science of Chinese medicine, acupuncture is an energy therapy designed

to create balance and harmony in your body. The therapy includes puncturing the client's skin using many pin-shaped needles and strategically placing them along various meridian points in the body. Using these meridian points, acupuncture is meant to help the client's internal energy re-balance and re-calibrate so they can live healthier lives. Acupuncture can treat various issues, including headaches, back pain, joint pain, fibromyalgia, and women who are experiencing labor pains. When we experience physical pain, it is usually because our internal energy is imbalanced; therefore, it manifests into physical pain. Alleviating this pain helps you experience internal and external healing.
- **Therapeutic Touch:** Encouraged relaxation and serenity are some benefits of therapeutic touch. With it, you can improve your sleep hygiene, hasten the healing process after surgery, or reduce muscle pain. Stress and anxiety can also be managed with its help.
- **Healing Touch:** Like therapeutic touch, this energy therapy promotes harmony and helps re-calibrate your energy to experience natural healing. During a session, practitioners use their hands to connect with the client's energy and manipulate the flow within the nervous system so powerful healing can be felt.

Nature

Grounding yourself on the earth is an extraordinary way to raise your vibration. There is nothing like connecting to a natural energy source, such as taking a walk in the park or going for a hike. You get some exercise, and you change your vibration.

When connecting to nature, leaving your gadgets and artificial power sources behind is essential. Take this moment to reconnect with yourself, getting balanced in a more excellent state of consciousness. Do not let your cell phone take away your focus on the abundance and beauty that surrounds you in the present moment.

Taking a stroll or spending some moments in the backyard can make you feel better, more alive, and happier. Especially after a fight with your better half, when your kids are being difficult, or when work is stressing you out, immersing yourself in the beauty of nature can instantly shift your mood.

Yoga

Taking a consistent and mindful approach to yoga can help you nourish your body, calm your mind, and become more aware of the present moment. It is not just what happens in the external world that matters but also how you choose to react to it: yoga encourages intentional actions that prioritize health and well-being. Find inner peace through yoga; remember that the outside world does not decide your fate.

Some people will participate in yoga when they are in a low vibrational mood, such as when they feel anxious or stressed. Likewise, it can help calm their mind and give them peace and freedom from negative energy.

Moreover, yoga focuses on realigning your chakras. There are seven energy centers in our body, known as the chakras: *root chakra, crown chakra, throat chakra, heart chakra, sacral chakra, solar plexus, and third eye chakra.* Each chakra focuses on the part of the body from the inside out. For example, the heart chakra aligns your heart with a sense of purpose, love, and compassion so you feel fulfilled. The throat chakra helps open your throat so you can share your voice and message with the world. Yet, if one or all of these are out of balance, you can feel anxious, worried, closed off, stressed, and fearful, which are all part of low vibe energy. Practicing yoga moves helps realign and balance all seven chakras so you can feel more positive and raise your vibration by feeling a sense of peace, joy, harmony, and fulfillment.

Healthy Relationships

Surround yourself with people who embody positive energy, peace, happiness, fulfillment, purposefulness, intention, and gratitude; these relationships are essential for helping to increase your vibration. All of these elements add up to high vibrational energy; when you foster these qualities in those around you, your emotional frequency will be elevated too.

Jim Rohn says, *"You are the average of the five people you spend your time with the most" (Groth, 2012)*. When you think about this statement, ask yourself: *Are they consistently negative? Do they curse a lot? Do they gossip or complain? Do they constantly procrastinate and feel unmotivated or uninspired? Are they prideful?*

Becoming conscious of the attitudes and behaviors you display day-to-day is necessary. If your circle is full of disempowering negativity, it could be time to reevaluate who you choose to hang around with. To raise your vibration, seek out positive, like-minded people. People with ambitions, dreams, and goals; those passionate about success. Find those authentically happy with a meaningful purpose and feeling fulfilled, as these people will bring more positive energy and help elevate your vibration.

Take a break from all the arguments with your loved ones and spend some time alone or go for a walk. That way, you can reset your energy, attitude, and mood. Conflict brings low vibrational feelings, such as anger, guilt, and shame. Shifting your mindset and changing your environment, even for a short time, can help lighten your mood and help you feel calm and peaceful. One of the most significant relationships you will ever have is your relationship with yourself. Nurturing and fostering that relationship is essential to remain healthy, fulfilled, and happy. When these emotions are a part of your life, you raise your vibration instantly.

Restore Your Surroundings

This intention is so simple yet incredibly effective. As you can see from this pillar, raising your vibration does not have to be complicated; it is the littlest steps that make a big difference.

Taking care of your surroundings is a decisive action. By taking care of the environment you live and breathe in every day, you let go of what no longer serves you and clean up your habits. Not only does this affect your physical well-being, but it also benefits your mental and spiritual health.

There are a few ways you can restore your surroundings:

- **Clean out your purse or briefcase.** This may sound simple, but it makes a world of difference. Get rid of the garbage that does not need to be there, such as the receipts you no longer need and the documents that no longer serve a purpose. Tidying up these compartments can help you feel peace and a breath of fresh air, which can help raise your vibration.

- **Clean out your wallet.** It has been said that by cleaning out your wallet, you open your wallet to receive more abundance. If you think about it, this makes sense. *How could you receive more money if your wallet is messy and dirty?* This sends a message to the universe that you do not care about your current abundance. But by cleaning out your purse, abundance has a personal invitation to show up in your life and bank account.
- **Tidy up your home.** When your environment looks and feels unorganized and is a mess, it lowers your vibration. You feel grumpy, annoyed, frustrated, depressed, sad, and anxious. By taking a few moments daily or weekly to organize your home, especially your bedroom and office, you will mentally feel better, which helps raise your vibration.
- **Get better sleep.** 25% of our lifetime is spent in our bedroom, dreaming the night away. Having proper sleep hygiene is a crucial step in raising your vibration. When you sleep badly, you feel exhausted, tired, burned out, annoyed, grumpy, overwhelmed, lack concentration and energy, and unmotivated, which is not the right energy to start your day. Yet, implementing proper sleep hygiene makes you feel alive, excited, energetic, restored, and mentally healthy. You can practice proper sleep hygiene in the following ways: *turn off all technology at a set time, relax your mindset by reading a book or having tea before bed, put your phone on do not disturb or silent mode, meditate, say a prayer, and go*

to bed consistently at a reasonable hour, ensuring you get at least eight hours sleep each night.

Now that we have discussed the importance of raising our vibration and focusing on the positive things that life offers, our next pillar will discuss the importance of setting intentions. Being intentional helps you remain focused and steadfast in your goals and dreams. When it comes to manifestation, the intention is a crucial component of success.

Pillar Four
Intention

By definition, intention means the *"purpose or attitude toward the effect of one's actions" (dictionary.com, 2019).*

Each day, we take action on something, such as waking up to go to work or deciding what to have for dinner tonight. Likewise, we take action every day to achieve our goals, whether we like it or not. Sometimes, if we are tired when we get home, we do not feel like making dinner, but we know that we have to eat. In this case, we have three choices: *make dinner at home, order takeout, or go out.* Either way, it is our duty to make sure that we have dinner, regardless of the action behind it.

However, there is a difference between taking action and being intentional about that specific action. Using the dinner example, we can have pop and chips for dinner, which would not be healthy for our bodies. On the other hand, we can be intentional about it and make a nutritious dinner of salmon, vegetable medley, and potatoes. With the latter, it is not only healthier for our bodies, but it is also delicious.

This pillar focuses on the difference between merely taking action out of obligation and deliberately pursuing action as the pivotal step toward reaching your aspirations. By grasping this distinction, you can set your manifestation goals with purpose, insight, and pure will. When you clearly understand what you intend to do, the journey is extraordinary.

Intention Manifestation

Bob Proctor says, *"What you think about, you bring about" (2017).* This is a perfect example of intention manifestation. Remember, when manifesting and attracting positive energy into your life, it is essential to focus on uplifting and positive thoughts rather than negative or destructive ones. As Proctor said, *"If you think negatively, you will attract negativity into your life."*

Proctor's sentiment says it all when it comes to being intentional. As such, let us assume that you want to lose weight. In terms of reaching any goal, especially weight loss, be willful as our subconscious minds often take in what we think and say. Likewise, it is essential to stay aware of the words used. Instead of telling yourself you are fat or do not want to gain weight, try to reframe those thoughts into something positive. What you ask for is what your subconscious will give you. Ergo, if you wish to avoid gaining weight, call on your mind power and focus instead on your fitness goals. That way, your subconscious will be more likely to help you achieve them rather than working against them.

Be Intentional with Your Subconscious Mind

A few things to understand about the subconscious mind when being intentional with what you are manifesting are these:

- **It loves what is familiar and dislikes what is unfamiliar.** Suppose that procrastination is usual to you, while self-motivation is not. In this case, getting out of procrastination can be an uphill battle, as your subconscious mind is hardwired to take you back to what you already know. To successfully break away from this cycle of procrastination, you must consciously encourage yourself and make self-motivation the new norm. Establishing healthy routines that excite and inspire you will also help build up your motivation so that, eventually, procrastinating becomes a thing of the past. With consistent encouragement, you will find yourself more focused on your projects and better able to fight off distractions.

- **It does not understand past or future tense; it only understands the present moment.** When setting intentions for your manifestations, remember that your subconscious interprets only what you tell. Subsequently, when you say, *"I will no longer live in scarcity or lack,"* your subconscious may think this is precisely what you want and do everything to ensure that is the case. But if you shift your words and say, *"I live in enough every single day,"* the subconscious mind will believe that you are already living in abundance and will bring more opportunities for abundance.
- **It thinks with images and words.** Referring to the weight loss example, if you tell yourself that you no longer want to be overweight, all the subconscious sees are that you desire to gain weight and will present opportunities for you to earn extra pounds. Hence, when visualizing your dreams in your mind, you must visualize them in a positive manner rather than in a negative tone, as whatever you envision, you will attract.

When being intentional with your manifestations, be mindful of the words you tell yourself and the images you think about. Anything, positive or negative, will manifest as long as you think about it. A little thought-peep can say, *"I hope I do not lose my job,"* and suddenly, you are out of a job. Manifestation requires intentionality and staying mindful. Otherwise, all your subconscious can discern is scarcity and lack. This leads to it attempting to keep you in this state, as it presumes that is your aim.

To show the power of intention when manifesting, I will share a story about a woman who desperately wanted to get married and make herself happy but unfortunately went through some miserable relationships. Intending to achieve unconditional love finally, she replaced wanting marriage with simply wanting to get engaged. So, instead of telling herself, "I want to get married," she kept saying, "I want to get engaged." Besides that, she put a picture of an engaged couple with a beautiful diamond ring on her vision board. Then, a few years later, she mentioned at the seminar has been close to walking down the aisle multiple times, yet with each attempt, the engagement fell through before marriage which happened almost ten times. This illustrates how, when it comes to manifestation, your words speak louder than you may think to your subconscious mind.

How to Become More Intentional

There are many ways to become more intentional when manifesting your dreams. Here are a few you can put into action right away:

- **Vision board.** Making a vision board is a powerful way to express your desires and determine what you want to manifest. It enables you to become purposeful in noting what you dream of. As previously mentioned, it is essential to be intentional with your thoughts and words when creating your vision board. Suppose you want to bring about an intimate marriage. From there, incorporate images and phrases describing the relationship you wish for. If you dream of having $100,000 in the bank, include visuals illustrating people who already have this amount in their accounts. There are no set rules for making a vision board; make it your own. You can design it on your computer and make it the desktop background or lock screen on all your devices and enjoy looking at it daily. Alternatively, you can use construction paper, glue, and other supplies for a more traditional approach. Another option is making a movie version of the vision board, then watching it daily to embed the words and pictures into your subconsciousness. Let go of expectations; trust that this visualization will bring about all you want.

- **Journal.** Become intentional with what you are writing about. Speak of your dreams, aspirations, and goals. Get clear on your purpose and your passions. Give your dreams life by speaking into them as though they were already happening. Jot down what your higher self is saying in your journal and assess where any blocks may stem from to help you move on past them and find freedom. Other than that, there is a journaling strategy called scripting that can aid you in honing in on precisely what it looks like to live your desired life. Write everything out in the present tense and include info such as who you are with, where you are living, and the type of food you eat, as if you were in that very moment

living the life of your dreams. This method offers excellent clarity for visualizing exactly which dream life you would like yours to look like.
- **Say affirmations daily.** When you speak to yourself, make sure it is with uplifting and empowering words that are positive and in the present tense. By doing so, your subconscious will believe them and help you achieve whatever you want. For instance, if you desire to lose weight, remind yourself that you have a healthy and beautiful body. Likewise, eat nutritious meals daily that make you feel happy, lean, and gorgeous. The more positive statements you give yourself consistently, the nearer you will be to reaching your desired outcome.

Setting Intentions

Now that we have discussed how to become more intentional when manifesting your dreams, it is time to discuss how to set intentions and the importance of setting them, so you reach success.

By setting intentions, you can focus more on your goals and gain insight into what you hope to manifest. It is more than saying, "I want to have hundred thousand dollars in my bank account"; it goes beyond that. Intention-setting requires purpose, positivity, and commitment to ensure it is done correctly. To ensure your intentions are set with the right intention and vibes, it is essential to be aware of the attitude and behavior you are taking on while setting them. Additionally, having a real plan or structure for how your intentions will come to fruition can help give you direction so that you stay focused on achieving them.

Amina AlTai, a leadership and mindset coach, says, *"Intentions are an opportunity to design and take ownership of our lived experience; they are like setting the GPS for our lives"* (Estrada, 2022). By setting our intentions, we can effectively take control of our lives. It is like drawing up a roadmap to success; we can identify where we are and chart the course to our desired destination.

To set intentions successfully, you need to focus on the following information.

Know Your Destination

Get a clear vision of what you want to achieve. Ask yourself: *What is it that I want to bring into reality? A beautiful home? An amazing car? An unforgettable trip? A prosperous marriage? An incredible business?*

Whatever you desire to manifest, make it clear that you know where you are going. By setting intentions, you become purposeful with your destination. As such, instead of wishing for financial abundance, focus on what it would feel like to be financially secure. Affirm that you are already wealthy; visualize having $100,000 in your bank account, many clients, and feeling excited, blessed, and grateful. Doing this clarifies where you want to go with your wealth and sets you on the path to success.

Understand Your Why

You may be clear on what you want to manifest, *but why do you want it? What is the sentimental value you are attaching to your goals? Do you want thousands of dollars in your bank account so you can create remarkable experiences with your family and travel the world? Or is it because you want to become a philanthropist and give back to your community or favorite charity because it speaks to your heart?*

There should always be a reason behind every intentional action we set forth in our lives. When we understand these reasons, we will remain steadfast in our goals and be focused entirely on achieving them.

Focus on Who You Need to Be

Understand who the person is that has thousands of dollars in their bank account every month. *How do they dress? What do they do every single day? What are their goals and dreams? Who are they as a leader? What is their character like? How do they behave around others? Who do they surround themselves with? How do they speak? Do they speak with class, sophistication, and eloquence? How do they present themselves?*

By getting clear on the person you need to become that has manifested your dreams into reality, you know how to step into that persona. Start by releasing any blockages that keep you stuck. Focus on reducing the amount of cursing, as this type of low-vibe energy can be damaging. Analyze who you surround yourself with and look for more positive influences and networks. Re-evaluate your habits, stop procrastination, and become mindful of your choices. Once you focus more on the person you need to become rather than the person you no longer want to be, setting intentions will feel easier to accomplish.

Shift Your Mindset

Setting your sights on a target and focusing on the ways to get there starts the process of making your dreams come true. Instead of constantly striving, concentrate on being what you want. Give yourself an optimistic outlook, say positive things to yourself, convert negative ideas into supportive affirmations, be thankful for what you have already, and concentrate on what you intend to do rather than why it may not happen.

Have you ever heard the phrase, *"What if it works?"* It can be a game changer in terms of your outlook on life. Instead of worrying about failure, you can focus on optimism and possibility. By changing your mindset to this positive question, you will discover new ways to look at your dreams and goals with newfound confidence. This attitude shift is immediate and decisive, as it can help open doors previously closed due to fear.

Other than that, allow yourself to take the time to understand any limiting beliefs that keep resurfacing in your life by journaling them. Embrace a positive mindset and discover how it can help unlock potential you may not have known. See what changes can be made, and watch as they play out in your day-to-day reality. Writing them down and clarifying why they exist will help you become consciously aware of them, giving you the power to debunk them and shift your mindset to more empowering beliefs.

Be Consistent

One of the key ingredients to successfully setting intentions is to focus on consistency. Be dedicated and steadfast with your goals to accomplish them in no time. Clarity will help keep your focus and will help keep your dedication and perseverance intact.

For example, if you want to have a toned and fit body, you first need to be clear with your 'why.' Why do you want to achieve this? Is it because you want to live a healthy and active lifestyle? It is because you want to have a beach-ready body by summertime? Being clear about your goal will help you identify the specific steps you need to achieve it. That level of clarity can push you to remain consistent every day, no matter what.

Surrender Your Intentions

Being on the path of intention can be a demanding venture. When setting goals, you might feel alone, anxious, and pessimistic about bringing your dreams to fruition. Meanwhile, internal obstacles can come from doubt, procrastination, or losing enthusiasm. Not to mention convincing yourself that your manifestations would not come true because you have not seen tangible evidence yet. That said, it is noteworthy to remember that even if it feels lonely and stressful, having an optimistic mindset is always crucial.

Moreover, asking the universe for help is necessary to make your manifestations come true. Your spiritual team is always on hand to guide you through whatever journey lies ahead. Put your intentions out there and surrender them, do not cling too firmly to what you hope will happen, but keep in mind that the universe could surprise you with something different. To make sure your goals become a reality, trust the universe and let go of any attachment to the outcome; this will bring a greater sense of peace, joy, and satisfaction.

Subsequently, you must relinquish control when surrendering your intentions. So often, when we manifest, we become attached to the outcome that it becomes a block to something far greater than what we had initially envisioned. And when they do not show up as we intended, we become disappointed, upset, and stressed, which brings us into a low energetic state. By remaining focused and open and surrendering our intentions to the universe, we can feel excited knowing that the universe is partnering with us to make our dreams happen.

Overall, achieving a beautiful and abundant life starts with knowing your goals and desires. So, setting clear intentions is the key to bringing your manifestations to life. Meanwhile, visualization is an integral part of this pillar, so we will now take a deeper dive into it. Hence, in pillar five, we will be devoted to this topic discussed earlier.

Pillar Five
Visualization

During pillar four, we spoke about the importance of setting intentions so you can become clear on what you want to manifest in your life. Setting intentions gives you the freedom to be, do, and have whatever your heart desires. Furthermore, with your thoughts and intentions, you can manifest as much or little as you desire. To attract the positive energy surrounding manifestation, maintaining a high-frequency state is essential. Hence, by setting clear action steps and aligning them with your desired outcomes, you will be able to stay in the right energetic vibration for the successful materialization of your dreams and ambitions.

In making the puzzle complete, visualization is the next piece you need. Once you have set your intentions and they have been made clear to you, the next step is focusing on delivering these intentions. In pillar four, I shared that the subconscious mind only responds to the images you think about and the words you tell yourself. As such, visualization exercises will help you become consciously aware of the images and the words you think about and will help you stay on track while remaining in a positive, energetic state.

Power of Visualization

Visualization becomes essential when it comes to success as it helps you use imaginative imagery to visualize succeeding at your goals before it even happens. Likewise, it becomes powerful in its own right because it enables you to use the creative side of your brain to envision your success and feel what it would feel like before your goals come to fruition. Feeling those emotions is part of high-vibe energy, so when you can get into that state of being, what you are manifesting becomes a reality.

Envisioning is like sowing seeds in the universe. By picturing in our minds, we sow the seeds of manifestation and signal to the universe our intention. The universe takes action by nurturing and providing what the seeds need to grow—rain. To ensure they reach their fullest potential, we must act consistently every day toward achieving our dreams. When they are ready, we can harvest them, reaping an abundance of rewards from our labor.

Meanwhile, we all have dreams that keep popping up in our minds, the ones we wish to make a reality. When we focus on them, actively visualize them, and believe they can be ours, it activates our brain's Reticular Activating System (RAS). This system is made up of cells that bridge our vision and manifestation, making them just one step away from being realized. For example, if you want to manifest driving a 2023 Tesla, include a picture of the car on your vision board, and visualize yourself driving one, your brain signals to your RAS that that is what you want. From there, you will notice Teslas parked in front of your house, which you have never seen before, stopped at a red light as you cross the street, in the grocery store parking lot—everywhere you seem to look, a Tesla is staring at you in the face. Then, your friend shares that they just bought a Tesla and asks if you want to take a ride. With all that, the universe seems to be answering your call; your RAS is getting piqued as if it says, "We heard you, and here is something coming your way."

The same goes for your dream vacation. As such, imagining a dream vacation in Hawaii can be inspiring. From looking at Airbnbs to researching the islands, it is easy to picture yourself sitting on the beach in Oahu, sipping a delicious drink from a coconut shell, gazing out at the ocean and palm trees. Likely, after you do that, you start seeing ads for Hawaii popping up on social media, hearing conversations about the destination on public transportation or around the office and getting emails about flight deals; all signs you are one step closer to booking your ticket.

When your RAS is activated and aware, pay attention to the signs the universe is giving you, as your RAS's mission is to motivate and inspire you to keep pining for your dreams. Also, it brings your dreams into your physical reality to show you that you have what it takes to make them officially yours. They may not be directly a part of your life, but your RAS demonstrates that indirectly they are. That said, you need to take inspired action to make them a part of your life rather than watch people around you manifest them. Likewise, this can also happen when we visualize experiences we do not want, so remember to be mindful of how you use your RAS.

Letting Go of What No Longer Serves You

Visualization also helps with one important thing: filtering out what no longer matters. By clarifying what you want, you begin letting go of the things that do not serve you or your dreams. As such, it helps you think and dream bigger than what you can envision for your life right now; there is no limit to what you can dream about. Likewise, visualizing helps you forget what is not meant to be a part of your dream and gives you something to look forward to.

For example, you may have two passions: photography and opening a non-profit organization. Maybe when you were a child, it was your dream to travel around the world, taking pictures of magnificent places. But as you grew older, you realized that your heart and service belong in the non-profit sector, especially since you noticed so many dogs and cats running around homeless on the streets. Due to that, you dream of opening up a shelter that will give them love, attention, and care, minimizing the number of homeless pets in your city.

By using visualization exercises, such as a vision board, you can filter out what distracts you from focusing on your current dream; that is the beauty of it. Likely, your dreams can change, and that is okay. As you let go of what no longer serves you, you filter out the excess distractions that steer you away from what matters most. Likewise, you send a message to your subconscious that you are clear on what you want to manifest, and now nothing will get in your way. Lowkey, it is as if you are making a solemn vow to yourself that you are in it for the long haul, no matter what.

Multi-Sensory Visualization

Sensory visualization is a profound topic. Initially, it may feel uneasy, as if people think you are crazy, and it may feel uncomfortable. However, it will feel extraordinary once you get the hang of it.

I am sure we have all heard of the book and the movie *The Secret*. The speakers in the film talk about *like attract like*, which is associated with the Law of Attraction, just as we discussed in pillar two. If you touch and feel it in your mind, what you manifest is already yours.

There is a part in the movie where a guy is sitting in his living room, flipping through a car magazine. He comes across his dream car and visualizes that it is already his. He closes his eyes and can feel the leather seats' smooth texture. He visualizes himself cruising through the city, waving to people passing by. He can feel it when he pushes the brake pedal and shifts and accelerates the gears. He looks excited, motivated, and positive.

This scene is a perfect example of multi-sensory visualization. It is about using all five senses to visualize your manifestations, so they become a part of your physical reality.

The Power of Visualizing with Your Senses

If you dream about that vacation to Hawaii, feel your fingers clicking the buttons as you book your tickets. Visualize yourself packing your swimsuit, flip-flops, shorts, and suntan lotion. Let your excitement flow as you tell your partner that you just booked the trip to Hawaii. When you are in the air, look at the blue sky out the plane's window as you descend toward the island. Observe the palm trees cascading in the background. Listen to the pilot on the intercom telling the passengers about the weather and that you are about to land, so you must put your seatbelt on and fasten your trays upright. Feel the sun's warmth basking in your face, ready to welcome you to the island. As you land, your ears pick up the voices of the locals saying "aloha" when you pass them on the streets. Careless the luggage handles between your fingers as you pull your luggage behind you. Savour the fresh coconut water in your mouth and smell the remnants of Hawaiian rum engulfing your nostrils. Touch the door handle between your fingers as you enter your ocean view room. Enjoy the ocean in the background as you look out the panoramic windows of your hotel room or step out onto the balcony. Take pleasure from the ocean breeze in your hair, the saltwater from the ocean, and the seagulls cawing above you as you look up into the sky.

Multi-sensory visualization is a powerful component of manifestation. It is what helps your desires become tangible. The more you hear, see, feel, taste, and smell in your dreams, the faster they will come to fruition.

Practicing Visualization

Visualizing your dreams is a fun, participatory journey. It is also a collaborative journey where you learn to partner with the universe. You decide what you want, and the universe reveals the steps to make it happen.

I encourage you to engage in a visualization exercise to practice manifesting to its fullest extent. Have fun with it and allow the universe to move through you so you can receive clarity on what you want.

To effectively visualize, there are a few steps to put into action.

Journal About What You Want

Write it all down. Try not to be vague. Be as specific as possible. It is important you use all five of your senses so you can truly get a feel of what you are manifesting. It would not be as effective if you said, *"I visualize myself driving my dream car. I feel excited about it."* There is no emotional response to this statement. It feels neutral. It feels as though if you get your dream car, great. If you do not, that is okay too.

But imagine if you were to say something like this: "I am manifesting driving my 2023 Tesla. It is a beautiful cherry red and has smooth, white leather seats. I can feel my excitement as I see it at the dealership. The moment I laid my eyes on it, I knew it was the one. I can feel myself sitting on the driver's side as I cruise down the streets. I can see my partner beside me, laughing and playing with the built-in touchscreen. I feel the wind blowing through my hair as my hands are on the steering wheel. I hear my kids laughing and having a good time in the backseat. I hear them asking where we are going, and I respond with, "Anywhere the wind takes us." As I stop at a red light, I can feel the smooth velocity of the brake pedals, and I can hear the engine roaring beneath me. I am excited and grateful as we stop at a local ice cream parlor for a delicious treat. I can hear the doors close behind me as I step out of the car, and I can feel my fingers push the button to activate the alarm and lock the doors."

Sensory visualization takes manifestation to a whole new level. When writing about it, write in as much detail as possible. Feel as though your dreams have already come to fruition.

Visualize Your Emotions

How will you feel when what you are manifesting becomes a reality? You can journal about this or simply close your eyes. Allow yourself to imagine how you would feel. *Would you feel excited about manifesting your dream vacation? Would you feel at peace knowing that you have manifested thousands of dollars in residual monthly income in your business? Would you feel joyful knowing you are now married to your soulmate partner? Would you feel grateful knowing that financial abundance flows into your life daily?*

By visualizing how you would feel when you reach your goals, you can feel one step closer. They can feel instantly tangible as if they are already a part of your life. Tapping into high-vibe emotions—such as happiness, abundance, gratitude, joy, and peace—when visualizing your dreams will allow you to feel the existence of your dreams before they physically manifest into reality. The more you feel about reaching your goals, the more you become motivated, determined, and inspired to make them happen.

Step into Action Consistently

Reaching your goals is more than a one-step process or get-rich-quick scheme. For instance, creating a beach body with toned abs and lean muscle requires consistent and determined action each day. It is not a one-time job; instead needs the courage to alter habits, strength, and determination to begin reaping the rewards of hard work. Sticking to nutritional meals, exercising at the gym regularly, keeping fit and healthy, avoiding unhealthy food choices, and taking accurate measurements in your diet can become a continuous cycle of motivated behavior and a process of consistent, clarified action.

To begin, you must understand why you want to manifest having a beach-ready body. If you are not clear, you will become unmotivated, which creates a lack of consistency. Sooner or later, you will wonder why you could not reach your goals. Yet, it is because remaining consistent became a struggle; therefore, you lost motivation. Despite that, consistency seems like a manageable obstacle when you know why you desire to manifest what you want.

Make Time to Visualize

More often than not, when people complain that their manifestations did not work, it is usually because they did not give themselves time to focus on them. Given that, make time to visualize your goals every day. In the previous point, we spoke about consistency, and this is the same thing. To become effective, visualize your goals a couple of times a day. Spend 10 to 20 minutes journaling or closing your eyes and envisioning what it feels like to live your dream life. Likewise, engage your five senses to feel, hear, see, taste, and smell your dreams. Allow yourself to feel what it would feel like when your manifestations are finally a part of your life. Wake up in the morning and spend some time visualizing while having some coffee. Get into the vibes of making them happen. Allow your subconscious mind to take in your visualizations. Create imagery and words in your mind and feel like they already exist. Before you go to bed each night, visualize your dreams again. Refrain from using technology, like playing games on your phone or checking your emails. Set aside this time for you and your goals.

Now that you can grasp the power of visualization and how it can help you manifest your dreams, the next pillar will set you up for success even further. This upcoming pillar will delve into the immense power of affirmations: *the words you express, both to yourself and out loud, possess tremendous strength.*

Pillar Six
Affirmations

Throughout this book, we have spoken about how our subconscious mind controls our life and decisions. Together, the unconscious mind and subconscious mind run about 95% of our mind *(Freud, 1915)*, so when we think about this, we wonder what is going on in the back of our mind to make us feel negative.

Affirmations are powerful in reframing our minds to believe more empowering beliefs. There is no doubt that your mind is a powerful tool. The words we tell ourselves can control our minds so strongly, thus affecting our behavior and decision-making.

This pillar will help you understand how powerful affirmations can be in your life. We will be discussing a few things:

- The importance of the thoughts and words we think and say.
- The importance of becoming self-aware of our words to ourselves and others.
- The importance of the words we say to the universe.
- The power of affirmations and how to write them effectively.

Understanding these key points, you will begin developing awareness of your actions, behaviors, and thoughts. Additionally, you will learn to notice what you are saying, how you are saying things, and how it emotionally affects yourself and others.

To manifest what you want, creating and practicing affirmations consistently will help you combat negative thoughts that disempower you. As such, they will help train and condition your mind for more positive beliefs so that, moving forward, you continue to empower yourself rather than tear yourself down.

The Power of Affirmations

Knowing how to transform your life starts with being mindful of the words the ones you say to yourself and those you share with others. Often, it is easy to overlook the power of such words when directed internally, so it can be surprising how much negativity we tell ourselves without even being aware of it. But awareness of our comments makes positive changes as our outlook is reflected in our lives.

Sometimes, we have moments when we feel like our lives are not going right and say things like, *"my life sucks."* But it is important to remember that the universe is listening, and it may take your words as affirmation that you want your situation to stay the same. You can feel frustrated at why nothing is changing even though you are trying to make a difference. To break out of this cycle, we need to be conscious of how much power our words have on our overall lifestyle.

For example, you could tell yourself, *"I am the Queen (King) of Procrastination"* every day. Although you may say this jokingly, your subconscious mind does not know the difference between a joke and truth; therefore, it will take your statement literally. From that, you constantly procrastinate when you try to work on a project with a deadline. As such, when you sit in front of the computer to work on the task that needs to be done, you find yourself playing game after game on your phone; hence, it seems that you have become exactly what you have repeatedly told yourself.

Ergo, pay attention to the words you say to yourself, as they have a powerful effect on your subconscious. Instead of using negative words, opt for positive ones. This way, you will shift your mindset and energy frequency to a higher vibration. In high-vibe energy, your positive manifestations start showing up in reality; *it is not 'magic,' but science.* And as you try speaking positively to yourself, you will experience its rewards.

Thoughts and Words Create Your Reality

The reality that you live in today is a reflection of your thoughts and beliefs. Hearing this can be challenging and upsetting but allow me to explain further. Every single aspect of your life has been shaped by the mental processes that you have gone through.

Think about it, *when we have negative feelings toward ourselves, what happens?* — we believe them. Our subconscious mind does not know the difference between positive and negative. It only knows of the present moment; therefore, it will believe whatever you tell it. If you tell yourself, *"I am not beautiful, and I will never find a good relationship,"* any relationship the universe brings you will not feel good enough. Your partner could treat you like royalty, but in your mind, you are thinking: *"Why are they even with me? I am not worth it. There are many other beautiful people they could be with. Why me?"* Due to this belief, your confidence and self-esteem are non-existent. Then the worst thing that could ever happen to you at this moment happens—they break up with you. In your mind, the breakup just affirmed that you are not beautiful, and you will never find a good relationship; otherwise, they would not have ended it.

Suppose you flip the situation around and think, *"I am so much to offer in a relationship. I am attractive, smart, and intelligent. My partner will love me for who I am".* Chances are that you will meet someone who cherishes you, and you give it your all. Interesting conversations flow naturally between the two of you, they express admiration for your beauty, and you feel confident taking their words as truth. This blossoming romance sees your self-love increase each day, and you are thankful for finding a partner who truly knows how to treat you right.

Norman Vincent Pale once said, *"Change your thoughts, and you change your world" (Zach, 2012).* Realizing that our beliefs shape our reality, it pays to be attentive to our words in our internal dialogue and find ways to turn disempowering ones into more positive statements. Our belief system is shaped by the time we are between zero and seven; what our parents say or do not say, how they behave, and the experiences they create for us become part of who we are. Thus, those same patterns may imprint on your psyche if you hear them speak negative thoughts or live out lack-based stories. Fortunately, with awareness and a new empowering mindset, we can break away from limiting thought patterns and create a completely different world. In short, choose better thoughts, and you will change your life.

Words You Say to Yourself

Let us face it; *we are often our own worst bullies.* In grade school, someone in your class threatened you with their intimidating behavior, bullying everyone they could find and putting everyone down. Unfortunately, you may have become a target of their aggressive tendencies, leading to derogatory names, physical bullying, and hurtful rumors. Childhood felt unbearable due to the bully's oppressive acts, leaving behind issues like depression, anxiety, and low self-esteem that you had to carry into adulthood. You believed whatever untruths were spoken against you due to this inevitable cycle of torment.

> *"You are a loser."*
> *"You suck."*
> *"No one will ever like you."*
> *"Your dreams are stupid."*
> *"You are ugly."*
> *"You are trying too hard. Stop being so desperate."*
> *"You are helpless."*

These words take a huge hit on your self-esteem. Many years later, you still believe these words, and your life is evidence that these statements are true. Now, imagine this is one bully from outside of you that made you feel this way. *What happens when you realize that there is an inner bully inside of you?* One that is stronger and more intimidating. As such, *do you know that self-talk has more impact than what someone who has gone from our lives might tell us?* It sinks right in if you look in the mirror and tell yourself you are not up to par and are not beautiful. However, if we express our uniqueness and loveliness to ourselves, we may initially be reluctant to believe it, but eventually, we do come around. Strangely enough, negative ideas are accepted more quickly than positive ones; negative thinking enters our minds easily due to our conditioning since childhood.

Look at the media; it portrays negativity every single day. Yet, cannot help but pay attention to them since it is all anyone ever talks about. Oddly enough, we rarely see uplifting stories covered by the media. When this was discussed, someone commented, *"Negativity makes the news, but positivity does not."* Taking this statement into account, the words you say to yourself matter. To manifest everything you want, you must start with the words you say to yourself. Our negative thoughts can get in the way; they are conditioned to do so regardless because they are what we are used to, but the trick is to become aware of them and shift them immediately. Rather than hang onto the belief that manifestation does not work, shift this and tell yourself better thoughts.

As I mentioned earlier, Tony Robbins quote, *"You cannot feel fear or anger while feeling gratitude at the same time" (2014)*. In other words, it is impossible to have negative thoughts and positive thoughts at the same time. You cannot say, *"I hate myself, but I love myself."* It just does not work. In fact, it sounds a bit silly when you say this statement out loud.

Since your thoughts and words create your reality, find a way to change your perception. A world-renowned hypnotherapist, Marisa Peer, says, *"Tell yourself a better lie" (2022)*. I want you to know something as I refer to this statement: *The negative anecdotes you tell yourself are false.* They are a lie you convey to protect from potential harm. Yet, your subconscious believes the negativity and stores it in the back of your mind to protect you. In this instance, this is where telling yourself a better lie comes in handy. As you shift your self-inflicting words, you may not believe them right now, but rather than tell yourself lies that are full of negativity and shame that block you from receiving what you want, you might as well shift your perspective and tell yourself an optimistic lie. At least it is full of empowerment and inspiration, and you will believe it to be true in time.

Words You Say to Others

There is a famous quote by Maya Angelou, *"People will forget what you said, people will forget what you did, but people will never forget how you made them feel" (Gallo, 2014)*. But with all due respect to Maya Angelou, I disagree with this statement. *Yes, people may not remember exactly what you said, but these words make them feel the way they do.* If you are having a conversation with someone and you are constantly degrading them and tearing them down, telling them that *"their ideas are stupid"* and *"no one will ever go for them,"* you can be sure that their subconscious mind will remember what you said and store these words for later use to help protect them from potential opportunities where this belief can rise. Your words will make them feel like they do not have anything good to offer the world, and they will experience sadness, worry, stress, anxiety, and, in extreme cases, depression. Subconsciously, they will remember your words for many, many years to come.

So, do your words matter to others? *Absolutely.* The words you say to others can either do two things:

- Make them feel good
- Tear them down

Paying attention to how we communicate is essential, not just with ourselves but also with others. A single derogatory remark can be damaging, eroding someone's self-worth and uniqueness. So, taking the time to consider our words is an invaluable practice that will help us cultivate meaningful and respectful relationships.

To help explain this further, here is a bit of a harsh example. *Full disclaimer, it is a trigger warning.* Referring to the bullying example in the previous section, we can all agree that some bullies are downright mean. They will say anything as a means to tear their victim apart. According to MedPage Today, Shannon Firth has said that teen suicide has jumped 29% within the past decade (2022). Adolescents who experience bullying double the likely cause of attempted suicide *(Hinduja & Patchin, 2019)*, which makes suicide the second leading cause of death for people 10 to 34 years old *(National Institute of Mental Health, 2022)*.

Our words can greatly impact how someone else feels; they can give strength or make somebody feel destroyed. That is why we need to be careful and think before we speak instead of acting impulsively. Unfortunately, it is too common to act first and reflect later; conversations like this can get us into trouble. And so I am sharing this example to demonstrate how powerful our words can be, especially when the other person may be emotionally vulnerable. Hence, take precautions in what we say so that the message we want to express is conveyed in a way that will empower the recipient rather than cause harm.

To be mindful, we can do a few things:

- **Take a deep breath before speaking.** When entering a heated discussion with someone close to you, take a deep breath. Before your words become a detriment to another's subconscious and self-esteem, take a few deep breaths before saying your following sentence. Taking the extra time will help you calm down and help make the conversation go smoother. This is called emotional intelligence.

- **Step away if needed.** To refrain from saying something you do not mean and needing to ask for forgiveness later, leave the room for a few moments. Go for a walk, step outside for some fresh air, retreat to your bedroom—take a moment to collect your thoughts. Doing so will calm your emotions, so you return to a neutral state of mind and then have a more constructive conversation.
- **Do not allow your emotions to drive your conversations.** Getting angry can make us say things to others we may later regret. That is why speaking from a place of neutrality rather than an emotional state is essential, as apologies and forgiveness become almost inevitable otherwise. Keeping a level head when engaging in conversation is critical to having productive discussions.

Words You Say to the Universe

As our words have extraordinary power to affect ourselves and others, they also send a message to the universe, stating our intentions.

> *"Every thought, feeling, word, and action you put forth is a memo to the universe."*
>
> *–Dr. Debra Reble*

Giving voice to negative thoughts and words can send subtle yet powerful messages to the universe. When you are running a business and, in a state of frustration, express an unwelcome wish like "I wish I did not have these clients anymore," even though it may be an emotional reaction, the universe will take it literally. Suddenly and almost as if by magic, your clients cancel their contracts, or their circumstances change, making it impossible to work with you. Likely, the universe grants your wish; you no longer have to deal with those clients. In response to your plea, you have been given what you asked for; your request has been heard.

> **"Unspoken and spoken words are among the most powerful energetic forces we have for co-creating our reality."**
> –*Dr. Rebel*

Whether you like it or not, you collaborate with the universe every day. Anything you think about, the universe hears. All you say, the universe listens. Your thoughts and words become your unspoken and spoken intention. They become the plans you co-create with the universe. You state the intention, whether positive or negative, and the universe does its job to comply with your request.

So, the next time you think or say something, consider that it may materialize into reality. Complaining about your job to everyone is not expressing gratitude or love. Love is one of the most powerful forces in the universe, and when you show love and appreciation, you receive more of those feelings back into your life. Just as hate or negativity brings the same energy back to you, it is indispensable to recognize how your words and actions reflect your relationship with the universe. You might be sending out messages that do not align with what you want in return; remain conscious of adjusting your attitude and behavior when conversing with the universe.

What Are Affirmations?

Affirmations are uplifting and empowering affirmations that, if said regularly, can bring about significant life changes. With words of encouragement, they help to battle and question negative thoughts. Using such powerful affirmations, one can change their existing limiting beliefs into more optimistic thought processes. For instance, start your day off with an empowering conversation of self-affirmations. Look in the mirror and focus on your strengths, accomplishments, and anything that puts a smile on your face. Choose words to warm your heart and set yourself up for success each morning. Practice repeating these positive affirmations, as they can lift you and brighten up even the toughest days.

Moreover, affirmations can be a great way to boost your abundance and self-love. When you recite positive statements to yourself, you start believing them and feel more confident. Despite this, many people are still uncertain if these affirmations help. And so, if your attempts at affirmations did not work out, the underlying reason could be one of two things:

- You are not saying the appropriate ones for your situation (we will discuss this in more detail in the next section).
- You are not allowing yourself to believe what you are saying because your negative thoughts and beliefs are taking precedence over the positive shifts; therefore, they feel stronger than changing your mind.

If this is how you have felt about affirmations in the past, knowing how to write them to transform your life will give you the confidence to have a breakthrough.

How to Write Affirmations

As we discuss this section, I want you to remember something: *your thoughts have the power to become self-fulfilling prophecies.* This is not magic; it is based on scientific research and studies demonstrating evidence that what we think, we become. Hence, what we think of becomes our reality.

When we question ourselves and ask, *"What if I fail?"* our minds can easily conjure up many ways to demonstrate why we are not succeeding. This evidence can be persuasive, making us believe that our thoughts about ourselves are true. Remarkably, these negative ideas come unbidden into our heads without us meaning them to. They become part of us due to being conditioned subconsciously to think they are facts. As we contemplate our musings, our subliminal mind duly searches for data near us to persuade us of their integrity.

However, what if we turn our thoughts around, such as not settling into negative thought patterns without conscious effort but intentionally choosing to amplify and cultivate uplifting ones? Likely, since our words and thoughts shape our life experiences, choosing to use language will bring you closer to your goals. Besides, affirmations are a powerful tool and can bring about invaluable change.

To write an affirmation statement that speaks to you and resonates with what you are currently struggling with, it is best to remember the areas you would like to change. An affirmation's effectiveness happens when you can focus on one issue at a time. By doing this, your subconscious can take note of it, and the universe can work to help bring the truth of the statement to your life. Below are a few points to keep in mind when creating your affirmations.

Focus on One Key Area

Any negative thought you can turn into a positive one. But it is important to focus on one area that you struggle with at a time. Once you have overcome it, you can move on to another issue. For example, *do you have a fear of public speaking? Do you desire to have an amazing relationship with a loving partner? Do you want to love yourself deeply and unconditionally? Do you struggle with losing weight?* Choose an area that you are deeply passionate about changing. When you know what that is, your subconscious mind will be open to changing it, and you will feel motivated to take consistent action. Your subconscious mind is conditioned to focus on only one area at a time, so make it count. As you believe what you are saying, you can add another affirmation for a different area of your life.

Choose a Realistic Goal

This is a vital aspect of affirmations. Not believing in what you say to yourself, your life will not change how you would like it to. Perhaps, it will feel like a never-ending journey; eventually, you may quit because you feel affirmations do not work. Yet, keep in mind that you must choose affirmations that work for your circumstances. For example, if you want to earn more money and currently make less than $1000, refrain from affirming that you want to make $100,000. Although this goal seems *"nice to have,"* it would not feel real. In your mind, it will feel like, *"Yeah, right. No way this can ever happen."* But if you affirm that you want to make $5,000, that will feel more achievable, and you will likely reach your goal in no time. So, if $100,000 is your ultimate goal, you can work your way up the ladder by starting with a simpler yet empowering goal with which your mind can get on board.

Release the Negative

For your affirmations to be effective, find a way to let go of the negative jargon that shows up in your mind. Journaling helps you do this. Think about how you want to feel and the outcome you want to get out of saying affirmations, and take notice of the negative statements that show up to combat your positivity.

> *"You are not good enough."*
> *"You are crazy to think your life can change."*
> *"That will never happen."*
> *"Stop lying to yourself."*
> *"Your life will always stay the same."*

Once you have written down all the negative statements, you can combat them with a positive comment. For example, *"I live a beautiful and abundant life every day," "I have the power to change my life anytime I want," "I am more than enough,"* and *"My life is being transformed every single day."* By reinforcing positive statements, you combat the negative, by, in the words of Marisa Peer, telling yourself a better lie.

Speak in Present Tense

In pillar four, we discussed that the subconscious mind only knows present-tense statements. Hence it does not know the difference between positive or negative and past and future. So, when creating your affirmations, speak in the present tense. Instead of saying, *"I will own my dream home,"* expressing something like *"My dream home is on its way to me"* will enforce a positive reaction. Likewise, writing your affirmations in the present tense becomes a self-fulfilling prophecy, as if you are tricking your mind into believing that you already have what you are manifesting. Thus, it will conspire with the universe to ensure it tangibly shows up.

Be Emotionally Connected

Creating affirmations to ensure a change in your life can be highly effective, but they only work if you have an emotional attachment. For instance, if you want to become a better public speaker, you can say, *"I am a confident speaker who wows my audience every time I step up on stage."* Feeling yourself saying these words can feel very exciting and motivating. Maybe it puts a smile on your face every time you visualize yourself on stage. However, not feeling emotionally attached to your affirmations will make them feel vague and unbelievable. Likewise, you will not feel motivated to continue. Your inner bully might even get in the way. Whereas, if you say an affirmation that brings meaning to your life when you think about it, it is bound to come to fruition.

Writing affirmations to help transform your life can be fun, empowering, and exciting. They are proven to help get you out of bed in the morning, ready to start your day with high-vibe energy. When you feel abundant, grateful, and full of joy, you see your manifestations come true. The final pillar is tying everything you have learned in this book to feel like your manifestation journey has succeeded.

Pillar Seven
The Process

Pillar seven, the last leg of the journey, is where we tie everything together. Everything that we have spoken about will all make sense.

It is one thing to think about manifesting your goals; it is another to put your efforts into action. So many of us get so pumped and motivated to change our lives, but when it comes to taking action, our goals seem to go to the back of our mind, and before we know it, our life remains the same. Usually, this happens because the hustle and bustle of day-to-day activities get in the way of our goals that do not feel achievable; therefore, we lose motivation. Think about new year's resolutions. On December 31, feeling excited, motivated, and energized, most of the world creates new year's resolutions. Then, as of January 1, they are ready to get rocking and make it their best year. Yet, a couple of months into the year, they are back to square one. They are no longer pumped, excited, or fueled with positive energy; instead, they are trying to keep their head above water, surviving through day-to-day obstacles. Then December 31 rolls around again, and the cycle repeats.

Certainly, you can say as many affirmations as you would like and get your mind on track, but your life will stay the same without any physical effort. The manifestation journey is a give-and-take energy; *you take action, and the rewards follow.* One key thing for success is a realistic strategy that is easy to follow and will keep you inspired. Often, when manifesting, we do not think about the steps to put in place, and at the end of the day, we are left with no rewards to reap.

On this pillar, the content will help keep you motivated and excited to begin your manifesting journey. The steps are easy to follow and will give you the clarity you need to keep going. As said throughout this book, the hardest thing is to remain consistent, especially when something needs to be fixed. Yet, this pillar will help alleviate your stress and worry and motivate you to continue working toward your goals.

Identify and Clarify

To manifest, you need to know what you want to manifest. Clarity and transparency are what will make the dream work. But when there is no clarity, there is no dream. *Sounds simple, right?*

Write down a list of things that you want. It can be anything. Allow yourself to dream truly. *What is it that you want to manifest? Your dream home? Is there a vacation you have wanted to take for years? Do you wish for a family of your own? Dreaming of having a loving partner to grow old with? Or do you want more clients in your business?* Whatever it is, get crystal clear on your desires. Understand why you want them. Allow yourself to be emotionally connected to them; this will keep you motivated and help you persevere.

As such, do not just say, *"I want to manifest my dream home because it sounds nice,"* as this statement does not sound motivating. Instead, say something like this, *"I want to manifest my dream home because I am excited to watch my children play in the backyard. I am excited to cook delicious meals in my state-of-the-art kitchen, host holiday dinners, and have hot cocoa by the fireplace. My dream home is where I will grow old with my partner while having sleepovers with our grandchildren. We will cuddle in bed, watch funny movies, and snack on popcorn. This dream home is where everyone calls it their home away from home."* With this statement, you will feel more excited to think about and inspired to achieve it. Thus, setting yourself up for success from the beginning of your manifestation journey is how you perceive your experience from the get-go and will determine your outcome.

On the other hand, *have you been trying to get clear about what you want for a while and have yet to be successful?* Not a problem. Asking yourself *why questions* will help; it is called the **Seven Levels Deep Exercise**. This exercise will help you gain clarity and should take a few minutes to complete. You can do it with as many of your desires as possible.

Here is how it was done: Start with one question and then answer it in your journal. Chances are, the first question will sound a bit vague and empty, but the trick is to keep expanding your answers as you continue asking yourself questions. Around the seventh question is when you will receive deep clarity about why you want to manifest something.

Take a look at how to do the exercise with our ideal home as an example.

1. **Why do you want to manifest your dream home?**

    I have wanted to manifest it for a while; it would be awesome to have it.

2. ***Why would having your dream home be awesome?***

   For most of my life, I have only been renting the homes I have lived in, so I would love to have a place I can call my own.

3. ***Why does having your home matter to you?***

   Having my own home feels like success to me. I would love to give my family the home they deserve, where we can live in it for a long time and create remarkable memories.

4. ***Why does this matter to you?***

   I would love to see my children raised on a property they can call their own. I am excited to watch them run around and play with their friends in the backyard. I am excited to see them bring friends for movie nights and sleepovers. I am looking forward to hosting Christmas for my family and decorating my house with a ton of festive decor. I am excited to cook dinner with my partner in the state-of-the-art kitchen we designed while having a glass of wine. Afterward, we cuddle on our oversized, white leather sectional with a fluffy blanket as we watch a movie on our 60-inch wall-mounted plasma TV. We tuck our kids into bed and then enjoy the rest of the evening together, basking in our love and feeling grateful for a place we can call home.

   The statements went from, *"I want to own a home because I think it would be awesome to have"* to *"I want to own a home because of the extraordinary experiences and memories we can create as a family."* Ergo, identifying what you want to manifest and getting clear on why you want to manifest it does not have to be rocket science. All that should matter if your manifestations are heart-centered and unique. And when you feel emotionally connected to what you want, the power returns to you.

Ask the Universe

The universe has your back, no matter what. Once you know what you want to manifest and why you want it, reach out to the universe. Ask for guidance from your spiritual team. You are always co-creating your life with them, so you must communicate with them consistently. And as a verse in the bible says, *"ask, and you shall receive."* However, if you do not ask, how can you receive anything? Sure, the universe can guess what you want, but if you are not clear with them from the beginning, it may give you something you did not expect or desire.

There are many ways you can communicate with the universe:

- Prayer
- Journaling (you can keep a spiritual journal, which contains your conversations with the universe)
- Meditation
- Visualization exercises
- Affirmations
- Manifestation rituals

Choose a way that resonates with you and be consistent with it. When you have clarity, you can share your thoughts with the universe and ask them to bring them to you, which will work to make it happen. Then, as you receive what you are asking for, you must also express gratitude to the universe for helping you bring it to fruition. Yet, being ungrateful, the universe may work slower to bring you other things. In essence, *why would they continue helping someone who is not grateful for what they receive?*

Take Inspired Action

If you want your manifestations to come to fruition, you must take action. Take steps toward achieving your goals. They do not have to be big steps; they can be small daily. For example, if you want to launch your first business and get clients, you must do more than sit around waiting for clients to come to you. First, identify why you want to launch your business. Then, you must conspire with the universe, tell your spiritual team what you want, and ask for it. Once that is done, you must create a website, launch your social media pages, and tell your audience what you are doing.

Staying motivated during the process and having fun are essential. However, procrastination will occur if you find that things are starting to feel tedious or lonely. That said, it is helpful to have affirmations ready as they will keep you on track. Plus, having a daily to-do list can help you stay on top of your commitments without becoming overwhelmed. Now, this checklist will help keep you inspired and on track to achieving your goals that day. As long as you hold yourself accountable for achieving your daily tasks, what you are manifesting will show up before you know it.

Trust the Journey

To truly conspire with the universe, you need to trust its guidance. Throughout your journey, there may be times you will feel like giving up because things are not working as quickly as you would like them to. This will feel frustrating, and you may feel disappointed and upset and believe that trying to manifest was a waste of time, and says, *"Nothing has happened yet, so clearly manifestation does not work."* With that said, the universe hears you loud and clear. Now, they are going to show you evidence of why you believe manifesting does not work and would not give you anything at all. And once again, you have proved that you could never achieve success.

This may sound all too familiar. Yet, here is something you need to know: *Even though it does not seem like anything is working, something is happening beneath the surface.* When we plant a seed, it takes a while for it to sprout. We nurture and care for the seed daily but cannot physically see it growing. Little do we know underneath the soil, the seed is growing inch by inch. Every time we nurture it, it grows even more until one day, when it is time, tiny leaf peaks through the dirt and out into the open.

Therefore, have faith in the process; your request to the universe has been heard, and you have its support to help nurture your seed until it blooms. If you struggle with complex or negative thoughts, remember your affirmations and say them until you feel content. Being in this tranquil state allows for further progress on your journey.

Release Attachment

As humans, we crave control in every aspect of our lives. If we somehow lose it, we feel defeated as we are not used to not getting our way one way or another.

Throughout the manifestation journey, it is effortless to get ahead of ourselves and hold a tight leash on the results. We want our dreams to show up in our physical reality so badly that we forget to have fun and enjoy the process. However, by not relinquishing control, you do not allow the universe to co-create with you. Due to that, it cannot work its magic in your life and show you the next steps if you have a tight grasp on the whole project. And so, you must learn to let go. Release attachment to the outcome and fully trust the universe and the plans they have for you.

Moreover, we all yearn to achieve our goals as quickly as possible, but sometimes this can leave us disappointed and discouraged if we do not get the desired outcome. Yet, by releasing expectations and trusting that whatever happens is for the best, we may find that our situation turns out better than we imagined. Taking the time to appreciate and enjoy the journey towards those goals rather than speeding through will ensure a much more fulfilling experience in life.

Be Grateful for What You Receive

Ego and pride get in the way of your manifestation journey. However, always express gratitude whenever you have reached your goal or are one step closer. Show appreciation to the universe for helping you move closer to calling in your manifestations. As such, if ego gets in the way, thinking that you succeeded alone and had no help from the universe or anyone else, you step back into low-vibe energy and forget about trusting the process. When that happens, it would not be surprising that things stop flowing your way.

Simply put, when you are grateful for what you currently have, the universe will give you more things to be thankful for. On the contrary, by allowing your pride to control your receiving, the universe will do what it can to keep you humble. Usually, that means pausing all abundance until gratitude becomes a part of your life again.

Overall, gratitude is one of the strongest emotions for effective manifestation. Think of it as being more grateful means receiving more. And to tap into a more grateful heart, here are some ways you can do:

- **Priming.** Every morning, you can do a priming meditation to set your day up for success. This exercise offers huge benefits as it gets you to think about all the things you are grateful for. They can be big or small. The first book you have published, meeting your partner, celebrating an anniversary, the birth of your children, the first day you got your new pet, the time you bumped into an old friend at a coffee shop, the time your partner surprised you with your dream vacation, the day you fell in love, the moment you visited Italy for the first time and sat in the Sistine Chapel—if you think about it, there are many things you can prime your heart to feel grateful for every morning.
- **Journaling.** Very similar to the priming exercise, but instead, you write down what you are grateful for. You can do journaling in the morning and evening if you wish. I encourage you to start small; begin with five or ten things. You can gradually increase to 20 or 30 and make your way up. Some of the most successful people in the world can think of over 100 things to be grateful for every day.
- **Focus on what you have now.** Be grateful for it. It could be watching your children grow up. The way your partner makes your coffee and brings it to you in bed every morning. The friends that call you regularly to see how you are doing. A steady paying job that helps you pay the bills every month. A success-

ful business brings in residual income and amazing clients every month. The clients who have already chosen to work with you. The car that brings you to work every single day. A warm house to keep you and your family safe and protected. The abundance of food you eat daily. When you acknowledge all you have now, the universe will continue bringing in more goodness.

Watch Your Energy

As you know, the Law of Attraction states, "like attracts like." Hence, take care of your energy during your manifestation journey, as you will receive the same energy you are showcasing to the universe. For instance, if you are always angry, frustrated, and annoyed that things are not working your way, the same energy will come flooding back to you. It will be evidence that manifestation does not work, your life will still feel like a mess, and it will feel like everyone you have ever loved is conspiring against you. You will feel like a victim, not a champion.

However, if you choose enlightenment, abundance, and gratitude instead, you will receive the same back tenfold. It will feel like your life is finally clicking into place; you will meet extraordinary people, your creativity will skyrocket, and you will feel motivated and inspired every day. Your life begins to transform because you are paying attention to your energy. Positive and negativity are like an energetic force field that tries to pull you in at any chance. Whatever you decide to gravitate toward will be up to you, but it will depend on how your energy is feeling.

If you are in a funk and you want to shift your energy instantly, here are some helpful tips:

- **Put on some dance music and move to the rhythm.** Dancing releases endorphins and gets your adrenaline pumping, which helps bring you into an immediate state of joy.
- **Watch a comedy.** Funny movies or shows bring out the laughter in you. Smiling (laughter) releases dopamine, endorphins, and serotonin, known as happy drugs.
- **Meditate.** Meditating will help you feel calm and relaxed when stressed and worried. Likewise, take a few deep breaths and say your affirmations while you are smiling.
- **Smile.** No doubt, smiling makes you instantly happy, especially if the person you are smiling at smiles back at you. In this situation, it feels like instant gratification and being authentically happy changes your life.
- **Sit up straight.** Your posture plays a big part in how you feel in every moment. If you are always slouching, you feel mentally, emotionally, and physically exhausted and wish for the day to be over. Besides that, it might even make you feel sad or alone. Being mindful of your posture can brighten your mood right away. Sitting up straight rather than arching your back makes you feel alive, alert, and motivated. Plus, it promotes a healthy spine, so it becomes a win-win.
- **Go for a walk.** Grounding yourself in Mother Nature can certainly put you in high-vibe energy. As such, it

promotes calm and stillness and helps bring peace to your mind, body, and spirit.

Let Go of Limiting Beliefs

When you have not received your desired results, ask yourself why. Perhaps, it could be because you are still holding onto some negativity blocking you and keeping you stuck. And with such negativity, you must clear the path so positivity can start flowing your way. Remember, *abundance cannot flow on a busy road*; you need to remove the resistance, so it does not get stuck trying to get to you.

There are a few steps to take to fully clear any negative distractions:

- **Acknowledgment.** Understand why limiting beliefs are a part of your life in the first place. *Are they protecting you from potential harm?* When you allow yourself to understand, you create a deeper relationship with yourself that is full of love and happiness.
- **Forgiveness.** Free yourself and others from instilling limiting beliefs in you. Let go of the past so it no longer harms your present or future.
- **Accountability.** *Do not play the victim; play victor.* Hold yourself accountable for adopting these limiting beliefs and negative thoughts, and forgive yourself for holding onto them for so long.
- **Embrace.** As you hold yourself accountable, embrace and accept all parts of you. Understand that your limiting beliefs may not leave your life for good, but feel grateful that they are around to demonstrate your resilience and determination.

- **Shift.** Reframe the negative thoughts. Create new and empowering beliefs that will uplift you and keep you humble.

Another thing you can do is to write yourself a letter. We spoke about this exercise briefly in pillar three. Following these steps, write a letter acknowledging why the limiting beliefs are lingering and express gratitude to them for keeping you safe up to this point. Make a promise to yourself that you will strive for a better life because that is who you are. Vow to yourself that you will do everything in your power to release the resistance that keeps you stuck so you can transform your life and habits into empowering ones that keep you motivated.

By following this process, you are guaranteed to manifest your dreams. It will take some time, so it is important to remember to trust the process and to call on the universe for guidance. Even if things are not showing up right away, that is okay. Allow things to flow and learn to balance your energy so you can feel abundant, prosperous, and authentically happy. When you can stay in this state, what you are manifesting comes to fruition effortlessly.

Conclusion

You have reached the end of the book. Congratulations! I hope you are proud of yourself for accomplishing this part of your journey.

We have covered many aspects to help you start your manifestation journey on the right path. I trust that you will take these pillars and develop your understanding of the subject matter in a way that relates to you and your situation.

The only way for us to learn is to grow, and by reaching the end of this book, you have grown on a deeper level, mentally, physically, and spiritually. Not everyone seeks to better themselves consistently, but by reading this book and applying the knowledge to your own life, you have taken the next step toward personal and professional growth.

We have covered many topics to help enlighten you on your path:

- **The origin and science behind manifestation.** By understanding this, you can get behind what it truly means to manifest your dreams.
- **The 12 spiritual laws of the universe.** By now, you understand that manifestation is not simply about the Law of Attraction. That is only one law out of twelve. I encourage you to use these laws to get what you truly desire out of life. Notice how they play into

your life, see which ones resonate with you, and then focus on them.
- **The importance of vibrating at a higher frequency.** The higher the energetic frequency you vibrate daily, the easier it is to manifest anything you want. Understanding how vibrating on a certain energetic frequency affects your life by changing extraordinarily.
- **The importance of gratitude** and how feeling grateful can change the trajectory of your life.
- **Why healthy relationships are essential and how they connect** to your manifestation journey with yourself and others.
- **Setting intentions for your goals is vital** so you know where you are going and how to get there.
- **Taking inspired action consistently** can improve your life (it is not just about the big steps!).
- **Why learning to co-create with the universe** can transform your life immediately.
- **The importance of visualizing your dreams** and how visualization techniques can help shift your subconscious mind into believing your dreams are possible.
- **The power of the words** you say to yourself, others, and the universe. Change your words, and you change your life!
- **How to create empowering affirmations** that can set you up for success.
- **Getting clear on the process** while having fun, watching your energy, and trusting the journey.

I intend to help you through a challenging phase in your life by writing this book. Maybe you are struggling financially or feeling stuck in a job you hate. Perhaps you wish to find a beautiful relationship or take that vacation you have longed for several years. Whatever you are currently going through, I have done my part by providing incredible solutions in this book that are guaranteed to change your life. I have shared a blueprint of what it takes to drastically change your life. Now it is up to you to take the next step: take action. Once you do, there is no doubt your life will transform, but without inspired action, your life will stay the same.

If you know someone who could also benefit from reading this book—your parents, friends, coworkers, cousins, siblings, your children's friend's parents—anyone that you know that is also struggling and would like to get their life back on track, I trust that you will share this book with them. This book can benefit anyone ready to make a drastic change in their life: Those prepared to go after their dreams and manifest them into reality. It is never too late to say yes to yourself and your dreams. Sharing this book with our loved ones, you help them experience freedom and healing.

Lastly, I encourage you to apply the knowledge you have learned on these pages to your life. If there is one thing I would like you to take away from this book, it would be this: You have the innate power in your mind to create extraordinary things. What we lack is the action that keeps us motivated and inspired. Applying this knowledge eliminates inaction and promotes inspired action. Action that makes us excited to get out of bed in the morning, with a smile on our face and pep in our step. Your manifestation journey begins the moment your thoughts form—create them wisely, and you will one day live the dream life you have envisioned.

Glossary

Affirmations: Positive and empowering statements, words, or phrases that are known to set you up for success; affirmations can be anything related to wealth, business, relationships, health, wellness, or spirituality. Usually begins in the form of an "I Am" statement.

Consistency: Taking action regularly to build a stable habit while focusing on your well-being.

Emotional Intelligence: Understanding how to regulate your emotions and balance them in the middle of certain situations so the outcome does not appear negative.

Emotional Regulation: Balancing your emotions so they do not affect your decision-making.

Gratitude: Demonstrating thankfulness in receipt of a gift, help, or service; acknowledging one's efforts and showing appreciation for how they have impacted your life.

Intention: A heart based plan that focuses on a goal or outcome.

Inspired Action: Setting yourself up for success by knowing and fully understanding why you want to manifest something and using those reasons to keep you motivated in reaching success

Journaling: Writing down your sentiments, thoughts, and feelings in a notebook on a particular subject to understand the root cause of an issue.

Law of Attraction: A philosophy dating back centuries that helps us understand the interconnection between our thoughts, actions, and behaviors.

Limiting Beliefs: A state of mind in your subconscious that, when perceived, can cause a negative impact on your life that results in feeling stuck, unmotivated, confused, and never moving forward.

Manifestation: The scientific process of visualizing something in your mind and turning it into a tangible person, place, or thing.

Meditation: A creative art form that helps you calm your mind, relax your body, and bring peace to your well-being. It can be in the form of music, sounds, or voice activation.

Multi-Sensory Visualization: Utilizing all five senses (see, hear, taste, touch, smell) to effectively visualize succeeding at your goal before it happens.

New Age Spirituality: A mixture of divine beliefs, both in a religious and spiritual context. People who follow new-age spirituality do not believe in one thing; they study different religions and engage in various spiritual practices.

Present Moment: Being aware and acknowledging what you have in your current surroundings; taking a moment to check in with yourself and your energy without getting distracted by technology and social media.

Releasing Attachment: Surrendering, having faith in the unknown and letting go so you can be open to an unexpected outcome.

Pseudoscience: A collection of practices disguised as part of scientific studies but don't appear to be factual or true.

Spirituality: Divinity; the belief that a greater power guides your path. Not based on religion; based on a cluster of beliefs.

Subconscious Mind: The facility in your mind that stores memories, experiences, and other information; often referred to as the mind's warehouse and makes up about 95% of the mind's capacity together with the unconscious mind.

Surrender: Having faith in the process and fully trusting the journey without a logical understanding of what will happen.

The Universe: A group of spiritual beings or entities who co-create with you to help transform your life.

Vibrational Being: A state of being; the energy you perceive in the universe.

Vibrational Frequency: The speed at which a human's energy is calculated. If you radiate negative energy—such as frustration, anger, and worry—your vibrational frequency is low. Meanwhile, your vibrational frequency is higher if you radiate positive energy—such as happiness, gratitude, joy, peace, and enlightenment.

Vision Board: A creative form of visualization. It can include magazine clippings, printed images and words, and colorful and unique ideas of how you want your life to be, a powerful manifestation technique.

Visualization: A manifestation technique that helps us think in imagery and words to clarify what we want.

References

Bob Proctor. (2017, April 27). AZ Quotes. https://www.azquotes.com/quote/805850

Borbala. (2017a, June 26). *5 ways to raise your vibration and have more positive energy (part 1).* Follow Your Own Rhythm. https://www.followyourownrhythm.com/blog-1/2017/6/18/5-ways-to-raise-your-vibration-and-have-more-positive-energy

Borbala. (2017b, July 10). *10 toxic habits that are lowering your vibration (part 2).* Follow Your Own Rhythm. https://www.followyourownrhythm.com/blog-1/2017/6/18/5bsh1ryhitjsknub-f47tnv1grtc6nq

Bradley, J. (2018, March 15). *Sensory visualization — A clear path to manifestation.* Medium. https://medium.com/@judestur/sensory-visualization-a-clear-path-to-manifestation-9461d8c01514

Brown, B. (2021a, October 4). *Law of Action | The 12 universal laws of manifestation.* Modern Manifestation. https://www.themodernmanifestation.com/post/law-of-action

Brown, B. (2021b, October 18). *Law of correspondence | The 12 universal laws of manifestation.* Modern Manifestation. https://www.themodernmanifestation.com/post/law-of-correspondence

Brown, B. (2021c, November 15). *Law of cause and effect | The 12 universal laws of manifestation*. Modern Manifestation. https://www.themodernmanifestation.com/post/law-of-cause-and-effect

Brown, B. (2021d, November 29). *Law of compensation | The 12 universal laws of manifestation*. Modern Manifestation. https://www.themodernmanifestation.com/post/law-of-compensation

Brown, B. (2021e, December 26). *Law of perpetual transmutation of energy | The 12 universal laws of manifestation*. Modern Manifestation. https://www.themodernmanifestation.com/post/law-of-perpetual-transmutation-of-energy

Brown, B. (2022a, January 23). *Law of relativity | The 12 universal laws of manifestation*. Modern Manifestation. https://www.themodernmanifestation.com/post/law-of-relativity

Brown, B. (2022b, February 6). *Law of rhythm | The 12 universal laws of manifestation*. Modern Manifestation. https://www.themodernmanifestation.com/post/law-of-rhythm#:~:text=let

Butterworth, E. (n.d). *New thought pioneers: Thomas Troward*. Truthunity.net. https://www.truthunity.net/courses/mark-hicks/background-of-new-thought/thomas-troward

Bullying, cyberbullying, & suicide statistics. (2020). Megan Meier Foundation. https://www.meganmeierfoundation.org/statistics

Cannon, M. (2015, December 14). *10 accidental scientific discoveries and breakthroughs*. InterFocus. https://www.mynewlab.com/blog/accidental-scientific-discoveries-and-breakthroughs/

Cronkleton, E. (2022, June 27). *Energy therapy: What to know.* Medical News Today. https://www.medicalnewstoday.com/articles/energy-therapy#uses

Davis, T. (2020, September 15). *What is manifestation? Science-based ways to manifest.* Psychology Today. https://www.psychologytoday.com/us/blog/click-here-happiness/202009/what-is-manifestation-science-based-ways-manifest

Davis, T. (n.d). *Manifestation: Definition, meaning, and how to do it.* Berkeley Well-Being Institute. https://www.berkeleywellbeing.com/manifestation.html

Duda. (2017, August 30). *What does Buddhism have to do with the law of attraction?* Little School Of Buddhism. https://littleschoolofbuddhism.kickassmuse.com/buddhism-law-attraction

Edison's Lightbulb. (2014, March 8). The Franklin Institute. https://www.fi.edu/history-resources/edisons-lightbulb#:~:text=In%20the%20period%20from%201878

Estrada, J. (2022, June 29). *Setting intentions are a "part practical, part magic" wellness practice, experts say.* The Zoe Report. https://www.thezoereport.com/wellness/how-to-set-intentions-for-manifestation

Filippazzo, F. (2021, January 4). *The Law of attraction: Energy, frequency and vibrations!* Medium. https://medium.com/know-thyself-heal-thyself/the-law-of-attraction-energy-frequency-and-vibrations-1d3fc438bbc1

Firth, S. (2022, October 12). *Teen suicides jump 29% over the past decade, report finds.* Medpage Today. https://www.medpagetoday.com/psychiatry/generalpsychiatry/101188

Forrest, L. (2007, November 28). *We are vibrational beings.* Lynne Forrest and Conscious Living Media. https://www.lynneforrest.com/spiritual-principles/vibrational-frequency/2007/11/we-are-vibrational-beings/

Freud's model of the human mind. (n.d). Journal Psych. https://journalpsyche.org/understanding-the-human-mind/

Gallo, C. (2014, May 31). *The Maya Angelou quote that will radically improve your business.* Forbes. https://www.forbes.com/sites/carminegallo/2014/05/31/the-maya-angelou-quote-that-will-radically-improve-your-business/?sh=5137d154118b

Goswami, P. (2021, September 28). *Vibrational energy and 9 ways to implement into your workplace culture.* Vantage Fit. https://www.vantagefit.io/blog/vibrational-energy/

Grasso, H. (2022, July 17). *The power of intention: 10 steps to manifesting your reality.* Gaia. https://www.gaia.com/article/the-power-of-manifestitation-10-steps-to-manifesting-your-reality

Groth, A. (2012, July 24). *You're the average of the five people you spend the most time with.* Business Insider. https://www.businessinsider.com/jim-rohn-youre-the-average-of-the-five-people-you-spend-the-most-time-with-2012-7

Guerin, N. (2015, July 20). *7 steps to manifest anything you want -- including money.* HuffPost. https://www.huffpost.com/entry/7-steps-to-manifest-anyth_b_7806936

Hay, L. (2014, November 26). *The power of affirmations.* Louise Hay. https://www.louisehay.com/the-power-of-affirmations/

Healthwise Staff. (2022a, January 3). *Healing Touch.* Myhealth.alberta.ca. https://myhealth.alberta.ca/Health/Pages/conditions.aspx?hwid=aa104487spec&lang=en-ca#acl6879

Healthwise Staff. (2022b, January 3). *Therapeutic Touch.* Myhealth.alberta.ca. https://myhealth.alberta.ca/Health/Pages/conditions.aspx?hwid=ag2078spec#:~:text=Therapeutic%20touch%20is%20based%20on

Hinduja, S. & Patchin, J. (2019, May 29). *School bullying rates increase by 35% from 2016 to 2019.* Cyberbullying Research Center.https://cyberbullying.org/school-bullying-rates-increase-by-35-from-2016-to-2019

Hurst, K. (2018, April 6). *The 12 spiritual laws of the universe and what they mean.* The Law of Attraction. https://thelawofattraction.com/12-spiritual-laws-universe/

Hurst, K. (2019, June 5). *Law of attraction history. The origins of the law of attraction uncovered.* The Law of Attraction. https://thelawofattraction.com/history-law-attraction-uncovered/

Intention definition & meaning. Dictionary.com. (2019). https://www.dictionary.com/browse/intention

Intermountain. (n.d). *Why it matters how you talk to yourself.* SelectHealth. https://selecthealth.org/blog/2019/05/why-it-matters-how-you-talk-to-yourself

Irven, J. (n.d). *19 ways to raise your vibration.* Sustainable Bliss Collective. https://www.sustainableblissco.com/journal/raising-your-vibration

John, H. (2019, September 25). *British Science Festival: 7 ways dancing can improve your life.* British Science Association. https://www.britishscienceassociation.org/blogs/bsa-blog/7-ways-dancing-can-improve-your-life#:~:text=Dance%20has%20been%20scientifically%20proven

Lieber. A. (2022, July 16). *The 7 major chakras: What you need to know and how to work with them.* DailyOM. https://www.dailyom.com/journal/the-7-major-chakras-what-you-need-to-know-and-how-to-work-with-them

Lopez, C. (2020, January 31). *The science behind good vibrations.* Balance. https://balance.media/good-vibrations/

Kurt, E. (2018, October 16). *2 high vibe drinks that will raise your vibration.* The Elegant Life. https://theelegantlife.com/manifesting-confidence/raise-your-vibration/

Mayo Clinic Staff. (2022, April 30). *Acupuncture.* Mayo Clinic. https://www.mayoclinic.org/tests-procedures/acupuncture/about/pac-20392763

McGinley, K. (2019, September 18). *How to Raise Your Emotional & Spiritual Vibration.* The Chopra Center. https://chopra.com/articles/a-complete-guide-to-raise-your-vibration

McLeod, S. (2015). *Freud and the unconscious mind.* Simply Psychology. https://www.simplypsychology.org/unconscious-mind.html

Mind Tools Content Team. (n.d.). *Using affirmations.* Mind Tools. https://www.mindtools.com/air49f4/using-affirmations

Moe, K. (2021, June 4). *5 visualization techniques to help you reach your goals.* Better Up. https://www.betterup.com/blog/visualization

Molitor, M. (2019, October 5). *The power of your brain | The 95-5% rule.* Linkedin. https://www.linkedin.com/pulse/95-5-rule-michele-molitor-cpcc-pcc-rtt-c-hyp?trk=portfolio_article-card_title

Mullins, E. (2008, August). *The process of the law of attraction and the 3rd law, Law of Allowing.* University of Wisconsin-Stout. http://www2.uwstout.edu/content/lib/thesis/2008/2008mullinse.pdf

Peer, M. (2022). *Tell Yourself a Better Lie: Use the power of Rapid Transformational Therapy to edit your story and rewrite your life.* RTT Press.

Potter, P. (2013, May 1). *Energy therapies in advanced practice oncology: An evidence-informed practice approach.* Journal of the Advanced Practitioner in Oncology 4(3). 139–151. https://www.ncbi.nlm.nih.gov/pmc/articles/PMC4093427/

Reble, D. (2017, January 19). *Words are powerful intentions to the universe.* Debra Reble. https://www.debrareble.com/words-powerful-intentions-universe/

Robbins, T. (n.d). *How the law of polarity can transform your life.* Tony Robbins. https://www.tonyrobbins.com/ask-tony/polarity/#:~:text=What%20is%20the%20law%20of

Robbins, T. (2014, October 31). *Tony Robbins quote.* Facebook. https://www.facebook.com/TonyRobbins/posts/the-antidote-to-fear-is-gratitude-the-antidote-to-anger-is-gratitude-you-cant-fe/10152793591744060/

Rollins, S. (2020, October 2). *The power of visualization: Improve your skill by training your mind.* Esports Healthcare. https://esportshealthcare.com/power-of-visualization/#:~:text=that%20way%20again.-

Rose, B. (2021, September). *The vibrational frequencies of the human body.* Research Gate. https://www.researchgate.net/publication/354326235_The_Vibrational_Frequencies_of_the_Human_Body

Scott, E. (2022, November 7). *What is the law of attraction?* Verywell Mind. https://www.verywellmind.com/understanding-and-using-the-law-of-attraction-3144808

Shahnawaz, G. (2021, July 8). *How yoga raises our vibration.* My Name is Ghanwa. https://www.mynameisghanwa.com/post/how-yoga-raises-our-vibration

Smith, S. (2023, January 24) *What does the bible say about manifestation?* Openbible.info. https://www.openbible.info/topics/manifestation

Spiritual Counseling Training: Intention manifestation. (n.d). Universal Class. https://www.universalclass.com/articles/spirituality/spiritual-counseling-training-intention-manifestation.htm#:~:text=What%20is%20intention%20manifestation%3F

Stanborough, R. (2020, November 13). *What is vibrational energy? Definition, benefits & more.* Heathline. https://www.healthline.com/health/vibrational-energy

Suicide. (2022, June). National Institute of Mental Health. https://www.nimh.nih.gov/health/statistics/suicide

Taleszia. (2018, April 14). *Top 10 foods for raising your vibration.* Happy Earth People. https://happyearthpeople.com/2018/04/14/top-10-foods-for-raising-your-vibration/

Vibrational energy - an overview,. (2013). ScienceDirect. https://www.sciencedirect.com/topics/chemistry/vibrational-energy

Vilhauer, J. (2020, September 27). *How your thinking creates your reality* | Psychology Today. https://www.psychologytoday.com/us/blog/living-forward/202009/how-your-thinking-creates-your reality

Wayne Dyer Quotes. (n.d.). BrainyQuote. https://www.brainyquote.com/quotes/wayne_dyer_384143

Who discovered electricity? (2019, May 11). Wonderopolis. https://www.wonderopolis.org/wonder/who-discovered-electricity

Wilinski, A. (2017, January 30). *Choose wisely: How our words impact others.* Brain Injury Services. https://braininjurysvcs.org/choose-wisely-how-our-words-impact-others/

Wolchover, N. & Leggett, J. (2021, December 22). *Top 10 inventions that changed the world.* Live Science. https://www.livescience.com/33749-top-10-inventions-changed-world.html

Wong, K. (2023, January 18). *What is the law of vibration and how to use it.* The Millenial Grind. https://millennial-grind.com/how-to-use-the-law-of-vibration-to-manifest/

World Smile Day - How smiling affects your brain. (2017, October 6). Aultman. https://aultman.org/blog/caring-for-you/world-smile-day-how-smiling-affects-your-brain/#/

Zach. (2012, March 9). *"Change your thoughts, and you change your world...".* Zach Mercurio. https://www.zachmercurio.com/2012/03/change-your-thoughts-and-you-change-your-world/#:~:text=Norman%20Vincent%20Peale%20once%20wrote

Zapata, K. (2022, July 22). *Exactly how to manifest anything you want or desire.* Oprah Daily. https://www.oprahdaily.com/life/a30244004/how-to-manifest-anything/

Made in United States
North Haven, CT
02 December 2023

44900273R00075